LABOURS OF LOVE

LABOURS OF LOVE

True Stories of Childbirth
in parents' own words

Foreword by
Sheila Kitzinger

Edited by
Dawn Robinson-Walsh & Jo Stewart

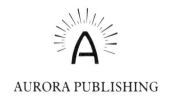

AURORA PUBLISHING

First published in Great Britain in 1993 by
Aurora Publishing
Unit 9c Bradley Fold Industrial Estate
Radcliffe Moor Road, Bradley Fold
Bolton, Lancashire BL2 6RT

ISBN 1 85926 000 4

Origination by
MetraDisc Limited
Rochdale OL11 3DT England

Produced by
PDH Book Print Production
Castleton, Rochdale OL11 2XD England
Telephone: 0706 711444   Facsimile: 0706 345557

Printed in Singapore

CONTENTS

Dedicated to:-

Jemma, Jamie, Camilla and Angus — may they be children at heart forever.

To Andrew and our wonderful joint productions, Alexandra Jennie and Laurence Stephen.

Our thanks to:-

Stanley Dutton, photographer for cover photo Tel: 0453 884438.

Jessica Winstone for lending her beautiful son, Benjamin, for the cover photograph.

Sheila Kitzinger for encouragement and criticism.

Jo Prowse, NCT Teachers' Panel, for helpful advice.

All contributing parents for their invaluable experiences.

INTRODUCTION

This is the book we both wished was available during our previous pregnancies – a book not of the mechanics of birth but about how giving birth really was for real-life parents. We hope we have selected a varied collection of reports from people from all walks of life who have undergone a variety of birth experiences, from the straightforward to the difficult, the exhilarating to the traumatic.

The book does not attempt to be medical or prescriptive (we are not qualified to take such a stance); we are not advocating or discouraging any particular practices and you will find women who have used all sorts of pain relief from relaxation and deep breathing through to epidural anaesthesia.

We hope that the book gives a truthful picture of what labour is like for individual parents, covers some of the issues which we approach with trepidation, and conveys a feeling of joy of the miracle that is the birth of a new life. You will see that no two births are the same but we hope that this book forms some part of a preparation for parenthood and a basis for parents to make informed choice in labour and childbirth.

The National Childbirth Trust

The National Childbirth Trust is Britain's best-known charity concerned with education for parenthood. It is run by, and for, parents through its network of 350 branches and groups.

This organisation offers help and support to members and non-members alike. There are a variety of services to help expectant parents choose the approach to pregnancy, birth and feeding best suited to them, and to provide guidance and encouragement to new parents. The services provided include Antenatal classes, Breastfeeding Counselling, Post-natal support, Post-natal exercise and discussion classes. The NCT also carries out research, resulting in an ability to offer better information to parents and health professionals regarding the opinions of both expectant couples and parents.

Antenatal Classes give parents the chance to become informed about all aspects of pregnancy, birth and life with a new baby. Relaxation, breathing techniques, massage and different birth positions are practised and explained enabling parents to approach the birth of their baby confidently.

Breastfeeding Counselling. The NCT actively promotes breastfeeding because of the many advantages it offers to mother and baby. There are over 500 NCT breastfeeding counsellors trained to help mothers establish and continue breastfeeding. They provide information and emotional support to help overcome problems and difficulties, enabling mother and baby to breastfeed for as long as they wish.

Post-natal Support. NCT's post-natal support system introduces new mothers and fathers to other parents and children in their area, giving them the opportunity to make new friends and share experiences. Special support is offered to those parents with more specific needs, such as working mothers, disabled parents and parents who have been bereaved.

Research, Education in schools, and Service on Local Health Committees.

The President, Eileen Hutton, and several NCT members contributed evidence to the House of Commons Select Committe on Maternity Services 1992 and the Consensus Conference 1993.

FOREWORD

*Most women expecting a baby are avid listeners
to other women's birth stories. They long to hear
about birth 'as it is,' with all the hope, fear,
pleasure, disappointment, the pain and the
striving, the triumph and delight.*

*This book is a rich source of information for
pregnant women and includes a wide variety of
accounts of birth experiences, telling how the
mothers, and the fathers, felt about labours that
were easy and difficult, straightforward and
complicated. Reading it will enable a woman to
develop her own rich anticipatory fantasies
about giving birth, and this is an important part
of preparing emotionally for a positive
experience.*

Sheila Kitzinger

STRAIGHTFORWARD LABOURS

Most deliveries are straightforward and we hope we have provided a variety of such reports. Birth, even where unproblematic, does not always go according to our plans and we include here a rapid first delivery and a long, posterior second labour. We have a father's report, and reports of vaginal birth after Caesarean and a vaginal breech birth. A couple of our reports detail problems with the delivery of the placenta following the baby's birth so are not strictly straightforward. One baby was born still in the amniotic sac (rumoured by old wives to be very lucky) and is a reminder that not all labours begin in the same way. This chapter does include one story where the parents later experience the death of their baby – we hope this, while a sad event, is related in a way which other bereaved parents find helpful.

DENISE
ORMOND

I read about other women's experiences during my pregnancy and found them awe inspiring, frightening and exciting at the same time. Being 33 when I had my baby I had many years to hear horror stories of labours and I was very anxious during my pregnancy but things worked out very well in the end. Perhaps my story will alleviate other future mums' worries that first births are long and painful. I know some are much longer but mine will redress the balance.

Apart from the need to rest at the end of my pregnancy due to high blood pressure, my pregnancy was quite straightforward. I suffered the usual early pregnancy sickness which wasn't three months but four, and not just morning but could last all day. I found nibbling snacks every few hours helped; bread especially was consumed dry at all hours. Alcohol was to be avoided at all costs to keep the queasiness at bay. Hearing of other people's sickness, I suppose I was fortunate that I was never actually sick and never missed any worktime.

I enjoyed certain things about being pregnant: being given seats more frequently on buses, longer nails than ever before and no monthly mood swings. However, no one prepared me for the emotional highs and lows one experiences as part of the tremendous hormonal body changes taking place. I would be weepy at the slightest thing on occasion and I remember weeping buckets in the bath one night as I stared at my ever increasing lump.

Attending antenatal classes with other couples helped to keep things in perspective and seeing the baby on the scan kept me going. I was getting prepared for a possible breech birth when the baby was lying sideways at 38 weeks. However, the head engaged soon after and I was most relieved. Because he was a long baby I was still getting kicks at the side as he was curled around. As I am nearly 6ft tall and my husband 6ft 4in we suspected a tall baby would be possible.

James was due on Saturday, November 2nd and after reading that only five per cent of babies arrive on THE day I was expecting to attend the local bonfire party. Perhaps a few rockets would set things off! But it was not to be. On Friday the 1st at lunchtime I had my show. There was no mistaking the sticky, pungent discharge which lasted a few hours. I felt nothing until bedtime when I began to experience a pain similar to a period pain. We went to bed but I spent a restless night as the pain grew stronger. About 10.00am I rang the hospital to see what I should do but was told to wait until the contractions grew more regular. The trouble was I felt a stabbing pain every now and then but not regular enough to time. I was never really sure if I was in labour so I kept up a normal easy Saturday routine.

My husband was with me all the time. The pains grew worse but I felt able to do some shopping in the afternoon. We didn't stay long as I was getting tired and the pain worsened. I was still not getting the contractions that I expected, just a dragging, more severe period pain. I was more comfortable kneeling with my head and arms slumped on a settee.

Sitting was more difficult. I had only eaten breakfast but not lunch and yet I was continually toilet trotting. On one of these visits about 4.30pm, the waters broke and there was no mistaking the sudden gush. The pain grew worse after that and we rang the hospital to say we would come in. I now experienced more of the contraction-type pain I had expected but it was more of a stabbing pain not a wave I had read of. We packed the final items quickly including frozen sandwiches for a hungry husband during a long labour.

The ride to hospital was uncomfortable and the babitens we had attached from about 4 o'clock was not very helpful. I should have been wearing it all day but not realising how far I was in the labour I had waited too long. When we arrived at the hospital about 6.00pm I couldn't wait to get on a bed. I was asked how frequent the contractions were but I explained, through gasps, we hadn't been counting as they were so irregular. The midwife told me they were every two minutes. She asked me to sign for Pethidine and I said I wanted to try gas and air soon. So I was given the mask. I was in the small admissions room as the other rooms were full.

By the time I had the monitor the midwife said she would give me an internal. She exclaimed, 'Good grief, you're 10 centimetres dilated'. I felt quite panicky at this point realising that the birth would soon take place. I expected at least 12 hours after arrival. We had no time to do our squatting or bathing, concentration or distraction exercises. I tried deep breathing and gas and air for a while before feeling the urge to push strongly. I told the midwife I didn't want a tear or a cut if possible and asked to deliver the head slowly. However, she soon told me an episiotomy would be necessary because he was a big baby. I didn't feel the cut and working at the pushing was easier than I expected.

One of my peers at work had said that the pushing was like being constipated with a melon and it certainly was a good comparison. I wasn't pushing long before suddenly the baby gushed out. It was a boy and the midwife exclaimed, 'look at his plates of meat' when she saw his large feet. He weighed in at 10lb 1oz and as soon as the cord was cut we held him and I breast fed him. Another midwife arrived to do the stitches and that was the most painful procedure of all. My husband held James and a second midwife held my hand and chatted to me while the stitching took place, but at least I had immediate stitches and was allowed to lie on the bed without wearing the stirrups I had seen on my hospital tour.

My husband was most put out that he hadn't been able to help with the positions and by the time James was delivered his sandwiches were still frozen!

See picture page 53

July 4th. Arrived home from work at about 5.30pm. Jane (my wife) was having pains which we presumed were contractions at hourly intervals. These pains had started at about 2.00pm that afternoon. We had our meal as usual but by 7.30pm Jane was becoming increasingly agitated and uncomfortable in both the standing and sitting position. She watched much of the England v. West Germany match (an indication that something must be wrong), on all fours supported on a bean bag. The contractions however were still what seemed to be a fair distance apart.

We went to bed at about 10.30–10.45pm and both admit to having slept well. Jane awoke wanting to go to the loo, which was nothing unusual, at about 1.40am. On arriving at the bottom of the stairs she informed me: 'I think my waters are breaking,' (I was relieved it hadn't happened in Tesco's). Rushing downstairs, I found Jane in the bathroom in deep distress. She felt weak, faint, sick and had the runs and I think she was in a state of shock. I managed to sit her down which she found very uncomfortable and then immediately rang the hospital to ask whether I should take her in. They asked a few questions and told me to bring her straightaway. I changed into some clothes, and was horrified to find that she thought her contractions were coming every few minutes. Fortunately the bulk of the items required for hopital had been packed in a case and had remained in the car for many weeks.

It took us twelve and a half minutes to get to hospital (not something I'm greatly proud of, but fear drove me on). I recollect little of what passed on that journey, but I remember trying to sound confident and in control in order to calm Jane. Whether it was my words or the movement of the car, I'm not sure which, but she was more in control of herself by the time we reached the hospital.

Our midwife was there to greet us at approximately 2.05am on July 5th. Any preconceptions about how the labour was going to go, what we would do, how we would sit, etc., were swept away by the pains of the contractions and the speed with which the labour was going.

Jane was linked to the monitor immediately in the delivery suite and so she got up and sat on the bed without hesitation. The pain she was in was already making it difficult for her to reason and the midwife offered Pethidine, which after waiting ten minutes, Jane agreed to have. Jane was four centimetres dilated when we arrived at the hospital.

I had taken up a position on the right of the bed, holding the

IAN NORTHCOTT

gas and air mask and looking across at the monitor on the other side of the bed. This position was certainly helpful, for it allowed me to provide gas and air whilst reading the contractions on the monitor thus helping Jane through them.

By 2.20am Jane accepted Pethidine and for the next half hour she contracted and yelled with what appeared to be anguish, and appeared extremely distressed. The Pethidine seemed to take effect at about 2.45am, and for the next three-quarters of an hour her contractions were dealt with, with more control.

The contractions were coming at about every 60–90 seconds and lasting about 30 seconds. Some were double peaks, which Jane thought lasted for ever. As the contractions intensified, so did the yelling fits. Jane also became increasingly agitated and distressed and requested to go home.

This frightened me, although I tried to hide it. However, the midwife was very perceptive and explained that Jane's emotional state was due a lot to the gas and air.

The contractions continued till about 4.30am, when the midwife asked if Jane wanted to push. Jane didn't seem to want to that badly, but pushed anyway (there was no transition stage, lucky for Jane).

Pushing was very tiring for her, but she did not appear to be in as much distress as with the first stage contractions. At about 5.00am, the midwife and I took a knee each, which Jane said didn't help very much, and she pushed against us. Her initial pushing was not long enough. Soon, however, with me breathing with her and a comment of, 'remember the grapefruit!', her pushing became more productive. She was tiring quickly. At 5.40am the head appeared which Jane didn't want to touch. By 5.55am the midwife informed Jane that with some good pushes the baby would be born by 6.00am. In fact, Jane did one almighty last push and Laura shot out at 6.02am.

The baby had gone into distress very near the end of the delivery and passed meconium. A doctor very quickly appeared on the scene to check her over following the cutting of the cord.

The memory of the seconds after Laura's birth are full of many thoughts, the most prominent being, is she alright and what a strange purple colour she is. The colour was a great surprise to me and might well have been off-putting if it hadn't been for the immense amount of activity that was taking place in the room at the time.

Soon after our arrival in the delivery suite, the midwife had asked Jane's opinion on episiotomy. At the time we had left it to her to assess its requirement. As she had felt Jane was tiring towards the end of the second stage, she had cut the perineum to assist the baby's birth. Following the satisfactory check of Laura by the doctor, I went to ring the grandparents whilst Jane received assistance in removing the placenta. She had an injection to make this come away, the midwife pulled the cord a couple of times and it came away in one piece. Jane said she was surprised at the size of it, she had expected it to be much smaller. When I returned about 5–10 minutes later, the placenta had been dealt with. Jane asked me if Laura Jane was an appropriate name and I agreed.

There followed one and a half hours of Jane being stitched up while I looked on, holding Laura Jane. This time was full of mixed emotions. Elation at the birth of a perfect new baby, fatigue and concern for Jane, who although she was receiving pain relief was still in a great deal of pain and asked the midwife if she was doing blanket stitch or cross stitch. I put this remark down to the gas and air, although the midwife didn't seem to take it personally.

By approx. 7.30am, the midwife went off shift, having stayed with us till the end, and we were left in the delivery room until about 9.00am when two very nice auxiliary nurses took Jane to have a bath. Following this we were transferred to the ward at about 9.30am. A quite incredible seven and a half hours had elapsed.

See picture page 55

VIVIENNE
HUGHES

Three thirty, Sunday afternoon, a week and a half past my due date: I have a show. Excitement. Should I page Richard? I'm not actually in labour, so I'll settle down to a session of gentle yoga instead.

Six o'clock: Richard arrives home, unpaged, and my contractions start immediately. They are regular, occur every five minutes and consist largely of backache. I kneel on the floor with my knees well apart, lean forward during contractions, sit back on my heels in between. No way can I walk around the house, make sandwiches, finish the ironing or do any of the things books suggest we use as distractions at the beginnings of labour. I know I ought to eat something. A plate of chips would be nice. Thank you, Richard, but I can't face the fish fingers you've cooked to go with them.

Nine o'clock: I feel it's time to make a move. Just one wrong number to a worried gentleman who assures me he isn't the maternity hospital, and then I am through. 'Are you coping with the contractions?', they ask. (With hind sight what an incredibly stupid question! If I'd waited until I couldn't cope, our baby would have been born on the lounge floor, ruining my Chinese rug in the process). I obediently follow the advice of, 'have a relaxing bath and come in in an hour or so.' This, incidentally, gives the mid-wives time to change shifts, but they don't tell me that.

I struggle up the stairs between contractions, struggle to get undressed, and struggle into the bath. There's not enough hot water in the tank for a very deep bath, so Richard starts a relay up and down stairs with kettles of water (neither of us think to fill the kettle in the bathroom and plug it in on the landing – rational thought has deserted us both). The bath is far too narrow for my kneeling position, while sitting on my backside makes the backache twenty times worse. By the third kettle, I have had enough. I struggle out, struggle to get dressed and struggle down the stairs.

I haven't seriously considered the possibility before, but suddenly I desperately want our child to be born at home. Driving off into the night to give birth in alien surroundings seems senseless. I say so to Richard – oddly enough he feels the same.

Too late however for that kind of decision now. If there is a next time, it will be different. I climb into the car and kneel up on the back seat. 'Aren't you going to put your seat belt on?' asks Richard. 'Certainly not, just drive.' Stunned disbelief. Doesn't he realise I'm in labour.

The contractions are very strong now. Breathing alone doesn't provide enough relief. I need to make a noise – not a gentle, breathy 'ah' or 'oh' suggested by my yoga tape, but something a little louder. The whole process is becoming more instinctive by the second. I wish I wasn't in a car being driven round twisty country lanes by an agitated father to be.

Ten-thirty. We arrive at the GP unit. Our midwife introduces herself, reads my birth plan and takes us to a delivery room. All very tasteful – floral curtains and grey carpet but not home. I drop to my knees and continue shrieking my way through contractions, now coming every two minutes. 'Oh dear they do sound painful', says the midwife, 'I'll do an internal in a bit and then we'll discuss pain relief.'

Pain relief? This woman is a midwife isn't she? Doesn't she realise shouting *is* pain relief? I don't need anything else yet. Except a mat, because the floor is pretty hard. I have to ask twice for the mat – I know they have them in the antenatal classroom. 'I'd rather you didn't actually give birth on the floor,' says the midwife once I've turned down her suggestion of kneeling on the bed. It seems a reasonable enough request and I foolishly agree.

She feels my tummy and predicts a boy. What? I'm going through all this for a boy? The baby is in the posterior position. This explains the backache, but at my last antenatal check it had been anterior. I mention this. 'Oh it's easy to mistake ROP for LOA,' she replies blithely, and being forbidden from mentioning Pethidine (I will ask for it if I need it, I have written on my birth plan) offers rectal chloride. 'What on earth is that?'. The mind boggles. 'Oh, a very old remedy.' Very likely, but I don't know its side effects so I decline. I am quite happy (for want of a better word) on my knees with Richard applying counter pressure to my spine at the peak of each contraction.

'Don't leap around so much,' instructs the midwife. 'You're ketotic already.' Hardly surprising really, considering the mammoth effort attempting to have a bath cost me. She suggests a glass of lucozade every half hour and I start to nibble on a Twix. She said 'already.' She can't think my labour very far advanced. Instinct tells me otherwise – I ask for an internal.

Eleven fifteen. I have an internal lying on my back on the bed accompanied by a contraction. It is the most painful part of the whole birth process. She is suitably amazed. 'This baby's turning really fast. And I can't feel any cervix at all.' I agree to have my waters broken. The warm gush is distinctly pleasurable. 'So it's OK to push is it?' I ask. 'I don't think you'll be able to stop yourself,' she replies.

At this point I had planned on squatting, but don't feel safe doing so on the bed. I kneel up instead and await the urge to push. Richard sprays my face with water after each contraction.

Ah bliss!

'How long till the baby's born?' I wonder.

'Oh it'll be here by two.' She clearly expects it to be before then as she calls in the auxiliary to watch the birth.

Two o'clock has come and gone and I am still waiting for the urge to push. The contractions are strong and frequent, but I'm not giving my uterus any help. I am using gas and air now. It seems quite helpful until Richard points out the blood on the mouthpiece – I'm not breathing the stuff in, simply biting on the mouthpiece for relief! So I take a deep breath and immediately feel giddy. I comment on this.

'That's not the gas and air, that's because you're hyperventilating,' she says. I'm not, but I don't feel like arguing.

Three thirty: the midwife is becoming agitated by the lack of a baby. She clicks the scissors around my nether end, intending to spur me on. Irritation. Why the rush? The baby isn't distressed, and neither am I. Richard, however, is wishing he'd brought earplugs.

'I'll give you a bit longer,' she declares after checking the baby's heartbeat, which sounds like a galloping horse.

Four thirty. She phones for my GP, then asks me to lie on my side so she can see if there's any reason for the baby to be stuck. There isn't. I decide I want to squat now.

'No, no stay on your side,' she says.

'No I want to get up.' This baby will never come out without gravity, or alternatively with my doctor on the way, an episiotomy and forceps.

'I can't see when you're kneeling,' she complains.

'I'll stand up then.' To her surprise (where am I getting the energy?) I do so and lean forward against the upright end of the delivery bed. This is better, and realising at last that I'm not pushing properly, she begins to school me.

'Chin on your chest. Don't shout – use the energy to bear down. Push. Again. Don't waste the contractions.' And then 'Put your hand down and feel the head.'

Amazement. The head is half out. 'How long's it been like that?'

'Ages.'

Anger. 'Why didn't you tell me?'

So I'm nearly there. I will get this baby born before my GP arrives. I'm getting the hang of this pushing now so why is Richard shouting 'Pant!' in my ear. Oh, I've done it! The head and arm are out, the tiny hand gripping the midwife's finger. It is six minutes before five. Another contraction and she is handing me my beautiful baby daughter, her large eyes wide and alert. Totally unfazed by the lengthy second stage, she scores nine on the APGAR scale and five minutes later, 10. The cord had stopped pulsating already. Richard takes three attempts to cut it. 'Are they always this gristly?' he complains.

I had expected to be emotional but am not. Knowing nothing about babies, ill at ease handling other peoples', holding my own is natural and right.

A few minutes later: the placenta arrives naturally, as per birth plan, but there is too much blood. I am given an injection of Syntometrine which stops the bleeding. I lie back exhausted while Richard cuddles our new daughter and our GP waltzes in.

He is quite happy (relieved?) not to be needed, checks the baby over and leaves. I start to bleed again. The auxiliary runs to see if the doctor is still about (he's not) while the midwife gives me an intravenous shot of Ergometrine. 'You may have a bruise later – your veins are collapsing.'

Sudden fear. I am no longer in control. How dare my body let me down like this? Thank goodness for the safety net of modern medicine.

Moments later: the bleeding has stopped. This cup of tea tastes delicious (I don't even like tea!). I am refused a bath but the auxiliary washes me down which comes a close second. On the ward: Richard is invited to stay as long as he wants. Our new baby is tucked into bed with me. Unable to sleep, we eye each other in wonder.

Stephanie Frances weighed in at a healthy 7lb 15^1/$_2$oz. I had no piles, and just a small tear that needed no stitching. I am eternally grateful to the midwife for allowing the second stage to go on for so long, though I feel it may have been shorter had I stayed on the floor. I am horrified to hear that the hospital may be facing closure – we need more low-tech GP units of this kind, not fewer.

ARABELLA LEWIS

According to the books, medical opinion and the majority of people's experience, most second labours are relatively quick and straightforward affairs. They usually last only a few hours. So we expected to go down to hospital and have the baby delivered very soon afterwards.

As it turned out we had plenty of time – thirty eight hours in total. The contractions began on Sunday afternoon and increased in frequency and intensity throughout the evening. Was this it or not? The week before I had spent all night at the hospital with intense contractions. The midwife said at 7.00am that we would see the baby in half an hour but then the contractions had stopped and I was told that nothing would happen. We realised later that in fact the pain was the baby changing from a posterior position to anterior. Since then I had been having contractions on and off. When my waters broke at quarter to one in the morning I thought that this was it – so off we went, again.

For the rest of the night the contractions increased rapidly and I felt able to cope by breathing. At 7.00am however my internal examination showed I was only two centimetres dilated. What was happening? Anyway after a lull the contractions built up again. My friend came in and gave me a metamorphic foot treatment which helped me relax and focus. However even though my GP came and after an examination said that the baby's head was engaged at six in the evening, another internal showed that there was no increase in dilation. This was in spite of contractions coming every minute and a half.

We were sent to the nearest city – there being nothing else that our local maternity hospital thought they could do. First we met a midwife from the wards, who sat and listened sympathetically and made us feel we were really being cared for. The decision was made to put me onto a Syntocinon drip from 9 o'clock. The idea was to enhance the contractions and promote dilation. So the night went on, with again much care and support from the next midwife, and of course Ralph. The midwife really thought she might be able to deliver me but she went off duty after having been with me all night without any sign of the baby. Before she changed shift an internal showed that there was still no increase in dilation.

Things looked very bleak and I felt very upset and disappointed. I was exhausted and we couldn't understand what was happening. We were both getting anxious about the baby – was there something wrong? On to our sixth midwife, who again was very loving and caring. I had no pain relief all night, at my choice, and was exhausted and drained as well as worrying about what was happening as the baby wasn't coming out.

At 9.30am the baby's heartbeat seemed to go down and everyone dashed in. A scan showed that the baby was OK but that her head was transverse. This meant that the crown was not presenting on the cervix so this might be one reason why dilation was not happening. My contractions were very intense and very frequent so the drip was switched off as my body had taken over. However it was suggested that if nothing had happened after another two hours then a Caesarian would be needed. I was on gas and air and felt a little spaced out. At about ten minutes past ten I felt the baby's head moving down. The midwife checked and there was the baby starting to come out. The cervix had dilated from about four centimetres to 10 in less than half an hour. At twenty past ten Ruth Eloise was born.

So after all that build-up and effort, a normal delivery which was very fast and uncomplicated. No-one could tell us why it was such an atypical second labour. Some suggestions were that the baby's head was not properly aligned or that the cervix had been resilient because of some trauma associated with the forceps delivery of our first baby! Of course we are sure that Ruth decided to take matters into her own hands after hearing the warning from the consultant. Whatever the reasons, Ralph and I see it as a process of shedding expectations and deepening the bond between us.

One thing that is certain is the gratitude due to all our midwives (six altogether) and the consultant who listened to our wishes in a very difficult situation. The NCT classes we attended were a source of great emotional and informational support. Ralph phoned our NCT teacher several times to ask what was happening and she offered many helpful ideas and cared.

See picture page 54

KATE

I was awaiting the birth of my second child with mixed impatience and apprehension. Although my ideal goal was to have a relatively active, natural birth, I had come to accept that I have a low pain threshold, so realistically decided that if this birth were to be as painful as the first I would opt for an epidural without delay or apology. I had heard and read many birth accounts which suggested it would be easier second time around. But also a few where the opposite was the case, so I felt hopeful rather than confident of a less gruelling labour. (The first baby had been induced two weeks early, with me immobilised by drips, monitor and an epidural which was only partly effective).

My second pregnancy was much more uncomfortable than the first; there were no serious problems but I felt plagued by a range of typical antenatal ailments, the worst being painful varicose veins in my thighs and vulva. It was no joke having to wear thick support tights through that long hot summer. I tried to comfort myself with the vague hope that as I had enjoyed a trouble-free first pregnancy, this unpleasant pregnancy might lead to a better birth.

Five days after my due date, when I was pessimistically starting to wonder if I was doomed to induction again, I awoke early feeling damp. Not having experienced the natural onset of labour before, I was unsure if this was a show or the waters breaking but a question and answer session by phone with the labour ward staff pointed to the former. There were vague aching sensations in my back but nothing like frequent contractions; however, it seemed best for my husband, Martin to stay at home. He and his two business partners had an urgent meeting scheduled for that morning which they held in our garden, while I waddled about the house pretending to be calm and even managing to do some of the relaxation exercises and breathing I had practised.

I had borrowed a TENS machine from the hospital and found it wonderful, not just because it was effective in distracting my mind from the pain while I breathed through contractions but also because it is completely under one's own control and unlike drugs does not affect the baby. I could not have coped with staying at home as long as I did without it. I spent the morning pottering around timing contractions with a stopwatch and imagining that I had a long day ahead as they were neither long nor regular, but I kept forgetting to time the intervals whilst adjusting the TENS knob and also trying to remember breathing techniques.

At about midday Martin's colleagues left and our two year old son Daniel went off surprisingly willingly with our friend on standby. I'd had enough of keeping active and retired upstairs to sit on a sofa with my electric fan, as it was yet another sweltering day. At this stage I made the mistake of relying on instructions to time contractions rather than on my own intuition about when to go to hospital. Now the pain was increasing and I was beginning to feel sick. I nobly or foolishly insisted that Martin should have his lunch and then we would leave, even though the waters now broke with a dramatic gush and the contractions were barely manageable any more. I felt unable to move and Martin was downstairs fixing his meal out of earshot of my feeble calls so I just turned the TENS level up and tried not to panic.

After a few very long minutes, Martin appeared and quickly disappeared again to get the car as near to the front door as possible. Somehow I faced the seemingly impossible stagger downstairs, and once in the car I could lean forward a bit, which helped. The traffic lights favoured us and my panicky feelings subsided as we approached the hospital. Having avoided the traffic jams we now faced the immovable obstacle of the maternity unit receptionist who seemed to find sorting out her filing cabinet a more urgent task than admitting me. I could hardly speak, let alone be persistent and assertive enough to demand action, so Martin came into his own at this point with the result that midwives materialised with a wheelchair to spare me any further hobbling steps.

By now half of me felt I could cope if I could just get on all fours to relieve the pain in my back, whereas the other half wanted an immediate epidural as I had been quite stoic enough by my standards. I told the midwife and student that I was going to give birth kneeling, which suddenly seemed not a matter of preference but an urgent instinct, as I was wrapped up in what was happening within me. So it was with great difficulty that they dragged my clothes off – it was too hot and hurried for modesty or hospital gowns – and persuaded me to get on my back for examination. My reward was to be told I was already over nine centimetres dilated and not far from pushing time so the bearing down sensations that necessitated the wheelchair had not been wishful thinking.

I babbled manically to Martin about how well I'd done without resorting to an epidural, and this elation enabled me to survive the transitional stage. It was all so fast that the midwives were still getting to grips with my medical notes when I needed them to check if I could start pushing, but I was at the point where pushing becomes involuntary anyway. I was doing what came naturally, which included shouting each out-breath despite being told to be quieter in case I didn't hear them tell me to stop pushing when the head appeared.

Three quarters of an hour after arriving at hospital the baby slithered out to meet us. He was immediately put in my arms but I was still on my knees trembling with muscle fatigue and couldn't trust myself to keep hold of this heavyweight. Ross Andrew weighed 9lb 11oz and was fit and well; I was fine apart from tearing, and felt incredulous that the kind of birth I had hardly dared hope for had really worked out.

My husband's role at the two births was different. I could not imagine the first without him to grip onto and groan into while the various machines and attendants did their work on me. In contrast, I felt in charge of the second birth, since the only technology involved was under my control, and I could choose my position. I was less dependent on Martin for direct comfort and support; instead, his encouragement enabled me to feel uninhibited and concentrate on my needs, while he acted as interpreter for the midwives when I was incoherent. In particular, he would have insisted on being able to deliver in my chosen position had we encountered an unwilling midwife. My experience certainly confirmed all I had read about upright positions speeding up delivery and easing back pains.

I had booked into the local GP unit at the hospital because I did not fancy the 'cattle market' situation at the hospital antenatal clinic. The GP unit offered two trips to the hospital, the rest at my local health care centre with the same two mid-wives and much more personalised care.

All went well until my 36 week appointment at the hospital was changed to 37 weeks. The baby was breech and time was short. The Consultant assumed I would want a Caesarean section with a week's stay in hospital. I tried to discuss an earlier discharge but he was adamant – I could not go home with stitches in. I knew other hospitals did discharge earlier but I did not seem to be able to get this through to him. I think he was surprised that someone would argue with him and not accept his word as law. As a nurse I was maybe less intimidated than others might have been.

When I discussed vaginal delivery with him, he was more helpful. My previous baby had been 8lb 1oz so he knew I could deliver a reasonable size baby. He agreed to pelvimetry to assess my pelvis which would have to be carried out the following week. I was so upset after that visit that I went to see my local midwife the next day who managed to reassure me and also said they would remove sutures. At 39 weeks I got the pelvimetry results: I could 'get a bus through' my pelvis, so it was agreed that I should try for a vaginal delivery with a section as a standby.

Unfortunately, the hospital does not have an epidural service except on a theatre list so I would have to have a general ana-esthetic. This time I felt I was able to talk to the Consultant, so I wondered if he had had a bad day the time before. There was also a group of student nurses all wanting to have a feel at the baby as a breech is unusual. It was interesting to be on the receiving end of teaching. The very supportive midwives in clinic advised me not to wait at home too long in labour in case of complications but otherwise to treat it as a normal delivery.

At 40 weeks and two days I awoke at 2.00am knowing I was in labour. We arrived at the labour unit at 6.00am to be greeted by the same midwife who had delivered our little boy, so we felt in safe hands. When she examined me, the sister thought my cervix was not dilated, but when I had a contraction it opened up well. She came to see me that night and said she had been able to feel the baby's heels but couldn't work out what they were. I had a drip put in just in case and a monitor attached. By the time the day midwife came on I was contracting every five minutes for one to two minutes at a time. Thanks to her I managed to breathe my way through the contractions. The Registrar (who would deliver the baby) and the Consultant came in on their way to the clinic

ALISON SPICER

and said they would call in later.

At about 8.15am I decided I would like some pain relief, so the midwife gowned up to examine me. Luckily she was beside me not in front because at that moment my waters burst and got the bottom of the bed. Out shot a foot and there was controlled panic. David my husband grabbed the drip and the top of the bed and I was pushed into the delivery room. All this time and as I somehow got onto the bed, the midwife had her hand over my vagina to keep the foot in. They tried to give me gas and air to stop me wanting to push but the tube was not long enough. A different Registrar arrived and complained that I had been in labour too long (he thought I had come in at 5.00pm) and why was I delivering vaginally? By this time he had gowned up and with a couple of pushes and a pull from him, our daughter was born at 8.42am. I knew forceps were often needed and episiotomies routine with breech babies, but I only had a slight graze. My only moment of panic was when – as we went into the delivery room – someone called for the paediatrician to be 'emergency bleeped'. Afterwards I realised they are there for all unusual births just in case. All our daughter needed was routine airway clearance and some oxygen and by 9.00am she was having her first feed.

The Consultant popped in on his way to clinic and was surprised at the speed of events. We were home in 24 hours as I had originally requested. Our health visitor thought there had been some mistake when she came as vaginal breech deliveries are unusual at this hospital, but thanks to very good midwives and the doctors at the hospital, a Consultant who agreed to try and, most of all a supporting husband, we had a normal birth.

The birth of our son Daniel, five years ago, although he was/is bright, healthy and beautiful, was rather a disaster. After some struggling we had arranged that he should be born at home, but when the time came he was a brow presentation, and after more than 36 hours labour, was so tightly wedged that he had to be pushed back up before he could be delivered by Caesarean! No-one seemed quite sure why all this had happened – although he was a big baby (8lb 12oz) I am also quite big – and the hospital where he was born had lost all our notes.

Four years on, before embarking on the next one, I hunted out the only doctor in town rumoured to do home confinements and asked if he would take me on. I knew no-one would consent to the next baby being born at home, but we thought that that was the best way to find a GP with the sort of ideas closest to ours. I had to agree to going into hospital, but the consultant agreed that I should have a trial of labour and that the birth should not be induced, etc., etc. I was, however, to ring up and go in the moment things started happening.

Things started happening a mere 12 days late (Daniel had been 18 days late, so we were all prepared for this) at about 1.00am on 26th July. I knew that the best way to stop labour is to go into hospital, so I turned over and went back to sleep, without even telling Nigel. I dreamed of squeezing through tight passages! Just before 7.00am there was a contraction strong enough to wake me – this time I woke Nigel. The next one came at 7.20am, and then at 10 minute intervals. They felt like the real thing but were not unduly uncomfortable. We still had no intention of telling the hospital – this is a labour report, not an advice manual. When I got up at 8.10am the contractions stopped and there was just the odd flutter. Dammit, we'd hoped they were serious because we were getting close to the limit on dates.

At 12.30pm we went back to bed to try a spot of natural induction. An hour later it worked – contractions were coming approximately 10 minutes apart and lasting about 45 seconds. At 7.00pm I had a show. By 7.30pm the contractions were stronger, lasting about a minute. Then Daniel, who had been with a friend, came home, needing food and attention – end of contractions! By 9.00pm though, they had resumed, more exactly 10 minutes apart, and lasting a minute. Still they weren't really at all painful, and I'm not sure how serious Nigel was taking them – I think he expected more theatricals! We asked if we could go in, find out what was really taking place – any dilation – and come home again if the answer was nothing; we were told not to worry and that we would know when it really was time to come in. However,

JUDITH MARTIN

by then I was sure things were speeding up, so we took Daniel back to the same marvellous friend and prepared to go into hospital – which I should have said is only about a quarter of a mile away, or we should not have been so relaxed. While I was getting my bag the phone rang – the hospital had looked up my file, found out about the previous delivery, hadn't I better get moving? We assured them we were on our way, and set off, rather expecting to have our knuckles rapped for behaving irresponsibly, not to say dishonestly, but our reception couldn't have been more charming.

However, it seemed they also expected more drama, and the doctor who was about to examine me said, 'It doesn't really sound as if you are in labour.' Our hearts sank as we felt now they've got us, they won't let us go, it'll be induction, that won't work, it'll be another Caesarean – but thankfully, I was two to three centimetres dilated. The sister took a blood sample, I declined an enema and all the other nasties, and we were left alone until 1.30am, contracting fairly erratically. Then we agreed to twenty minutes' worth of monitoring – you start to feel ungracious refusing everything. At least the monitor was a more civilised device than I'd had when Daniel was born, less intrusive, and the contractions weren't so bad that the belt was uncomfortable – and it was only for 20 minutes.

At 2.20am I had a bath, and Nigel washed his hair to boost morale for a long night! Then we both attempted to sleep, me on a hard narrow bed, Nigel in a chair – neither very relaxing. By 3.45am the contractions were too uncomfortable to ignore, and we gave up trying to sleep. We made the boring round of the labour unit, to pass the time and to help gravity. Some time around then I was slightly sick, and felt rather trembly. By 4.45am things were distinctly unpleasant, and I was sick again, though still able to make it to the bathroom. Contractions were coming seemingly continuously – I kept thinking, next time I'll have some gas and oxygen, it's too late this time, then when that one was over I was too exhausted to remember. In fact I suspect I dozed slightly between. Nigel said later that he'd have suggested gas and oxygen if he'd realised how far advanced I was – he'd been keeping it in reserve, so to speak, for when things got really bad! There wasn't time for any very controlled breathing; mostly I breathed deeply and occasionally remembered to go up to shallow breathing. I thought very sourly of Sheila Kitzinger, 'greet each contraction with joy . . .' Mostly I was aware that all this – not exactly pain, certainly not hard work (that implies something deliberate; I seemed to have no part in all this at all) – might still be for nothing, and we might still end up in the operating theatre. Then at 5.15am the sister examined me and said I was fully dilated — so all the really unpleasant bit had presumably been transition. Greatly relieved, but still not sure if we'd make it, we arrived in the delivery room at 5.30am, feeling bloody tired.

We'd asked in advance to have a try, at least, with the birthing chair. Then, it had looked very cold and hard, and a nurse said she'd bring pillows, but in fact it was beautifully cool. From about this stage, although I was uncomfortable, the thought of having to move or alter anything was unbearable. I felt no urge to push but was asked to do so — this accomplished nothing. Then at about 6.00am the urge came. The sister said the cord was around the baby's neck, though only loosely, and I had to pant. Events were pretty noisy by now — I had no urge to shriek or cry, but a good loud primal grunt seemed to help! At 6.07am, to my great astonishment, Rosamond was born. I'm not sure why, but I hadn't wanted to feel the top of her head when she crowned, and I didn't look down to see the head born — I didn't really believe any of it until she was all there, lying on me and not bothering to suck.

We'd asked not to have the routine shot of Syntometrine to expel the placenta, but the contractions had vanished for good and it did not appear. However, everything now was calm and quiet, the baby and I were cleaned up, she was weighed — 6lb 13^1/$_2$oz, a very sensible size — and we were just left together. At 7.45am the lovely sister who had been with us all along officially ended her night shift — and the placenta still had not been delivered. Much debate about whether to give Syntometrine now — by then I would have taken anything. The new sister arrived, although the other stayed, and had much less sympathy with these cranks — a swift yank and the afterbirth was out. Evidently it had not read all the books that say it follows naturally in about half an hour.

The conclusions that might be drawn from this are: a Caesarean birth doesn't have to mean that all others will be the same; that hospital staff are not all intransigent and unwilling, but it's still perhaps best to make any off-beat requests in advance, in writing; and, above all, don't go near a labour ward without your man — for hand-holding, face-wiping and general support, he's essential!

See picture page 57

DIANA BATTERSBY

Third child. Woke with a slight show, 10 days overdue. Contractions every 15 minutes throughout the morning – leant on walls, resisted pressure from my mother to go to hospital and played Trivial Pursuits. After lunch of tea and toast went to bed to escape mother! Dozed for half an hour or so and had to wake husband up at 3.00pm as contractions were stronger, now every 10 minutes.

4.30pm. Arrived at hospital, contractions every seven minutes and four centimetres dilated on internal examination. By 5.00pm I was esconced in a small labour room with own toilet, window open, and rocking chair to hand. Midwife had 'chosen' us because I wanted physiological third stage (ie, no Syntometrine). She had a very soft but reassuring voice, a competent approach (ie not always agreeing with us but giving her reasons) and was a member of Radical Midwives to boot. What luck! She would have used a birth chair if I had wanted but obviously wasn't keen as she said later that it was an inferior design and most women tore on it. We came to trust her professional judgement. I was belt monitored for 20 minutes – all well so it was removed. Later the baby was monitored externally with it which meant I only had the initial internal examination. I tried various positions. Problem with the rocking chair was that my husband couldn't rub my back and I was having severe back pains as the baby was, the midwife reckoned, probably facing my thigh. A step stool was excellent for squatting and kneeling while resting my arms on a pillow at the head of the bed. The wedge wasn't at all right for kneeling over. I found holding my husband was very comforting and I was very susceptible to his smell. If we'd had a double bed and less inhibition, I think we could have cuddled closer!

By 7.00pm, I'd lost track of time – contractions now every three minutes and lasting 45–60 seconds. Started gas and air. Communicated with husband by 'BACK' (rub) and 'FACE' (wipe). Pains in back becoming excruciating and I wanted only a fingertip caress but couldn't communicate this to my husband who was a bit bewildered by my stop-go policy on backrubbing. He told me times of contractions so I knew I was getting towards the end of first stage. Waters now feeling very uncomfortable towards end of a contraction. Midwife didn't do an internal because she felt she would pop them and possibly send me into unnecessary transition. I would have agreed to ARM or Pethidine at this stage but would have regretted it later. Midwife was attending a first time mother so we were usually on our own up to this point, feeling perfectly easy about it.

At 8.00pm I called for midwife as the Entonox wasn't affording enough relief and I was feeling a bit panicky as I knew I was too late for Pethidine. At 8.30pm (very aproximately) I suddenly decided I wanted to wee. This was my body taking over as I think it wanted a change of position, something my pain-preoccupied mind couldn't cope with. I can't remember if I did or not but the moving around helped my mental state even if getting back into the bed was an effort. I collapsed on to my side (having been previously squatting on a stool). The midwife then monitored the baby and the waters broke on the next contraction. 'Relief,' I remember saying, and immediately went into second stage with a hiccupy sort of contraction. This was disturbed by people coming and going as the shifts changed at 9.15pm and our midwife wanted a night midwife to witness birth to save her writing it up. I was taken aback by the severity of the pain and let out almighty groans. I was told to say less and push more and that if I relaxed into the pain (pushed it away) it would lessen. To my amazement it did. When the head was born, the midwife reminded Roy to flash the mirror about and I caught a glimpse of the head with the eyes open. Far more exciting was the soft wet feel of the head as I stretched my hand down. I panted the rest of the baby out and tore very slightly. The left lateral position which I had collapsed in was superb for the strong urges to push and I feel sure I would have really torn had I been squatting. The second stage was only five contractions, the last two for the head and body, and lasted 25 minutes. The 7lb 12oz boy was born at 9.25pm.

Then I sat and suckled the baby and waited for the placenta – and waited and waited. After 30 minutes the midwife advised Syntometrine and I agreed readily as I was starting to feel cold and shaky. At 10.15pm I delivered the placenta plus two large clots of blood which had been building up behind. Next day the midwife said she had been very worried as it was about 70–30 against the Syntometrine working at this late stage and the lovely birth would have been marred by a general anaesthetic. She was surprised that the injection had been necessary but it made me wonder if the risk had been worth it.

By 11.00pm I was ravenous, wanted a shower (disallowed) but went to the toilet on my own had no stitches and felt as fit as a flea! Our thanks to the midwife could not have been more effusive, more heartfelt.

Sadly, on 28th August, Guy died from viral pneumonitus at eight months.

Fourth child. 10.30pm. Finished gardening. Decided not to wash hair as I was swimming next day. Six days overdue.

2.30am. Woke with strong contraction. Mum said she had also woken at this time before I told her! By 3.00am decided I was in labour and would have to wash my hair after all. Wondered what I was playing at in the bath struggling with hair and contractions. Discovered I was 'leaking' whilst I dried.

4.00am. Called to Roy to wake up as I suddenly thought the birth may be imminent now my waters had gone. They had always gone at the end of first stage before. Mum got up, kettle went on. Emptied my bowels just before we left for the hospital – amazing how the body sorts itself out when left to its own devices.

4.30am. Hospital! Braced myself for all systems stop and indeed the rhythm went from the contractions which had been at five minute intervals. Porter insisted I sat in a wheelchair which put me in a black mood. You shouldn't have to fight bureaucracy whilst giving birth. Didn't particularly take to my midwife but felt she was trying to accommodate my wishes – she put us in a small labour room rather than the delivery suite. But she insisted I stay on the belt monitor because the baby's heartbeat wasn't recovering well after contractions. She would have liked the scalp monitor too but realised I was very strongly against it. It became apparent it was a busy night (twins born by section as I arrived) and I was very annoyed with hindsight that I had to suffer the constrictions of the belt monitor and be confined to bed because there weren't enough midwives to monitor me regularly. The belt monitor is just not a humane substitute for skilled care.

5.00am. I felt panicky when contractions stopped for over 10 minutes as I imagined they would start up super strong and unmanageable as they had with my second child. Roy suggested I 'tested' the gas and air and the midwife was puzzled when she entered to find me doing so between contractions. I felt calmer though uncomfortable on the bed. At this stage I thought I would shortly have the monitor off – had the labour been longer I think I might have insisted. I was four centimetres dilated on arrival so the midwife drifted in and out (more out than in). I concentrated on opening the cervix at the end of a contraction – imagining a kaleidoscope opening as the pain receded. It worked to my surprise. Occasionally, I felt quite high at the end of a contraction.

6.30am. Tried to get comfortable by sitting on a stepstool and leaning forward but I really wanted to walk, kneel and squat. Pain was quite severe now but I had time between contractions to relax and recover – unlike my first delivery. I declined the offer of pain relief and only took the gas and air spasmodically as contractions were uneven and I never knew until too late which the whoppers were. I suddenly felt sick – the midwife and my husband had been annoying with inconsequential chatter about dentists and pigeons but she wafted some air in my face and I felt better. I opened my eyes to see it was a grey disposable chamber pot which was wafting about and I felt (very vaguely) amused. She then left to deal with an admission and I felt cheated – I knew she knew I was in transition so why was she going at this difficult juncture. Sure enough, next contraction I wanted to push and asked Roy to press the bell.

6.45am. A strange 'nurse' in old fashioned hat and cuffs appeared but she couldn't do much. I had wanted the 'supported squat' but it seemed too much effort to get it organised (and too few people) so I lay on my side as the midwife had indicated earlier that she liked the left lateral position. The pain became dreadful and I could feel myself tensing against it. The monitor was appallingly uncomfortable now and I heard Roy ask if it could be taken off as the readings were unreliable as the baby moved. But no! Many contractions (10, 15, 20?) but little progress and I had pushed my third child out with three so I began to feel something was amiss.

7.15am. The midwife said she'd have to cut me on the next contraction as the baby was 'getting tired' – the heartbeat had dipped to 80 she said later. This heartened me as no one had said the baby was even visible so I was determined to get the baby out. As the contraction faded I carried on pushing like mad (never mind the pain, think of the stitches) as he eased out to my severe discomfort as the midwife tried to loop the cord from around his neck. I looked down and to my surprise saw the baby looking at me. Only later did I realise that it was him, and not me, the wrong way round!

7.21am, 21st July. Simon born! What joy! I had worried that Guy's death might have marred the birth but no – he was his own man. I loved holding him, feeding him, having my arms full again. Within the hour I was 'chaired' to the ward, enjoying a hot shower and awaiting admirers, bright eyed to start the day.

A tribute to Guy.

Fortunately, every birth report we received was a happy event with babies born healthily and most parents happy with the way events turned out. It does sometimes happen that a baby dies – sometimes at the end of a long illness, sometimes unexpectedly. This may happen during or shortly after birth or some months or years afterwards. Whenever and however it happens the death of a child is always devastating. We do not wish to dwell on this subject for too long in a book which is all about life, but felt that it was appropriate to mention Guy's death and to indeed offer a celebration of his short but remembered and very valuable life. Our many thanks to his parents for letting us use their reports.

On the sixth anniversary of your death:-

Today, your deathday, a letter came
asking for a poem about your birth, your life.
How could I describe in words your smile,
that unhurried happiness that you spread,
the memories of leaf-tugging that you left?

Again we return from holiday and the pile of towels
litters the hall. This time the children are older
and disappear to play with friends.
But your pram remains where the table now stands
and I see your rusk-stained reins empty still.

The brother you have never seen brings down his bears
and wants to play: leaves me no time to mourn.
But I remember, I remember, not the detail, not
the sounds, not the colours, but the joy you gave.
My tears fertilize a garden as the memories still fade.

Diana and Roy Battersby

We hope these words will bring comfort to any bereaved readers.

JO
STEWART

eptember 2nd. For seven days prior to birth, I had been discharging a very thick, jelly-like mucous. For two days prior to birth I had been 'uncomfortable' – in that if I stood still it felt like the world was going to drop out between my legs. Walking was fine, so I just didn't stand still. Worked hard Saturday and Sunday, got home 6.30pm on Sunday and went straight to put some washing in the machine. Noticed my 'birthing' night-shirt was amongst the things to wash, and as I bent to load it, a twinge in my back made me hope that I'd have long enough to get it dry! That was about 6.45pm, but at not quite 35 weeks I refused to believe that this was 'it'! During the evening, I had probably four or five cramp-like sensations, but decided I was just tired and achy. I took myself to bed at 10.30pm and decided a hot bath would cure all ills. From there to bed. During the night I woke most hours, either spontaneously in pain, or by my three year old demanding a drink. Each time I got up, I realised that I had extremely bad low-down back-ache, and forced myself to go back to sleep – I had set my heart on working right through the Wedding season – which finishes for me on 8 September – and with this baby officially due on 7th October, I thought I was safe.

Anyway, by 4.10am. I could no longer sleep for the pain. I woke Adrian and told him (I had not even hinted earlier, what a shokk for the poor man!) that I thought I was in labour. My first experience of childbirth had taken 12 hours, so I told Adrian, naively as it turns out, that there was no hurry and to go back to sleep.

Went downstairs, made a cup of tea and set about timing the contractions. They were coming every five minutes and lasting just over a minute, with occasional 'interim' ones, which meant there were long periods of time without any real break. By 4.45am they were so painful that I rang the hospital (totally unprepared – no phone number at hand!) – who advised me to come in. So, I woke Adrian again. He asked if there was any hurry, and I told him none at all, so he showered and made himself look devastating while I squatted on the landing panting and blowing! We rang my mother, who came to look after Jamie, and by 5.15am we were on our way.

By the time we'd reached the edge of town (20 minutes later), the pain was so intense that we had to stop on the side of the road for me to be sick. The pain was really low and severe, and the thought of another 12 hours of this terrified me.

And then we got lost. Had to ask two innocent bystanders for directions, found the hospital but couldn't find the 'rear, night-time maternity entrance' which we had been told to use!

Checked in at 5.50am, and we were shown into a delivery room. I sat cross-legged on the floor in agony until a midwife arrived. She was lovely – asked if I wanted to stay on the floor, or use the BirthDay bed which was in the room. I opted for the floor and she went off to find a mat while I changed into the night-shirt (which had dried in time). By the time she came back I was longing to push. I tried all the 'I must not push' and 'puff-puff-blow' routines, but the urge was too strong and I found it imposs-ible not to push. The midwife took a look, said she could see the head and that the baby was still in the amniotic sac, so that if I pushed gently we'd try and give birth without the trauma of breaking the waters. Eight gentle pushes and she was born, still in the sac, and 23 minutes after checking in! It was so easy I just couldn't believe it. The placenta was delivered easily and quickly without Syntometrine. I am so proud – no pain relief, no injec-tions, no episiotomy, no stitches.

Camilla weighed in at 6lb 5oz – huge for 34 weeks. She seems perfect – she was a little cold, but two hours under a hot lamp fixed that. She understood what a nipple was for from birth, so everything in our garden is rosy!

See picture page 57

Iattended the sub-fertility clinic before my first pregnancy – getting pregnant wasn't that easy! So after my son was born I wallowed in contentment, but although all my breast-feeding friends were rapidly losing pounds and inches, why wasn't I? Baby now eight months old – I was desperate – F-Plan diet activated. My jeans were still too tight and all I had was bran and wind. 'It's awful,' I told a friend, 'feels just like a baby kicking!' 'Maybe it is,' she replied. I was horrified, but knowing that breast-feeding wasn't an infallible contraceptive, off I went to the GP. My friend was right! Twenty-six weeks gone! I discarded the jeans for a voluminous dress and looked enormous!

I immediately enrolled at local NCT classes which were wonderful – the only time I had to think about this baby, with one of nine months already on my hands.

With no dates and a none too accurate scan, the next one was due on the 22nd, or the 9th, or 'sometime' in January. Christmas loomed, my husband was seriously ill with pneumonia, I had awful sinusitis and Sam had his presents out of a Sainsbury's carrier bag. Every night I went to bed, glanced at the carrycot space in the bedroom, and thought, please God, not tonight!

New Year came and we both felt better, the next night we were going out for a meal – our first celebration of the festive season. I paid the first of my thrice-nightly calls to the loo at 2.00am, went back to bed and soaked it (I had been going to put the plastic sheet on the next day). The midwife came, I had a bath, washed my hair, found a dry bed and went back to sleep.

Contractions started with a vengeance about noon – despatched number one to a friend and prepared lunch for the midwife and my husband. I found breathing as I had been taught in classes easy and a necessity and ended up spending contractions on all fours, as this eased the backache caused by the baby's posterior position.

At 1.45pm I told the midwife I thought I ought to go to hospital – she examined me and agreed as I was almost fully dilated.

I gathered my things together and got into the car, on my hands and knees still, but the front seat wouldn't go down with my ample rear behind it. The neighbours in our street were treated to a cabaret of my retreating out of the car on all fours and getting in the other side – we expected the police to be called to foil this kidnap attempt!

All the traffic lights seemed to be stuck on red and we arrived at the hospital at 2.30pm. One door said 'push', the other 'pull' – I knew which I needed.

The delivery suites were all full and my midwife was relieved I

MYRA JONES

had opted for a 'floor delivery', as this seemed all there was available. I availed myself of a very small room – not quite the broom cupboard – and not really having time to undress properly, I just popped Jonathan out.

My midwife was full of praise, not for me, but for my NCT teacher, who had obviously done such a good job in teaching me how to breathe and relax. Being on all fours had enabled the baby to turn from his posterior position.

I feel very priviledged, as I was an 'elderly overweight primip' and had two text-book pregnancies – not even feeling sick – or having any problems with blood pressure.

This was all five years ago, and it seems like yesterday. I felt very indebted to the NCT as I knew it was because I'd had such a good teacher that my second delivery had been so enjoyable.

From then on, I became very involved in the NCT, at coffee mornings, evening meetings and fund raising activities. I made many friends and became membership secretary and then secretary, trying to enable new mums to have the benefit of the same expertise that had made childbirth for me so wonderful.

On discovering that I was expecting our third baby, we decided that, as this would probably be the last, this time we would have the birth that we wanted, under water and as natural as we could. I had read about water births, and seen a television programme about it, and the idea seemed attractive – the thought of being able to be comfortable, the weightlessness and the lack of pressure appealed.

After discussing it with our GP we decided on a hospital birth due to the fact that both our other children had become distressed during second stage labour, the first narrowly escaping a forceps delivery after induction for failing to grow in the womb, and the second spending three days in the special care unit after a three hour second stage. However the local hospital was not impressed by the idea of a water birth, so the delivery was booked at a hospital several miles away where I used to work as a nurse and hoped for rather more support. At my booking-in appointment I saw the senior midwife who, although not discouraging, seemed to think it was just a silly idea I had got into my head, that I would probably forget about.

Despite this, the majority of the midwives were enthusiastic, and hoped all would go well. It was not to be at my next appointment at 28 weeks, I discovered that nothing had been done to make a water birth possible.

Meanwhile, I had contacted the Active Birth Centre, about hiring a birthing pool, and found that besides themselves, a company in Middlesex and one in Bristol, there were no other birthing pools to be hired. I thought then that I surely couldn't be the only person North of London to be interested in a water birth and after a lot of thought and discussion with my husband, I decided to buy a pool rather than hire one, and to try to hire it out myself. Back at the hospital, I found that the senior staff appeared to think a water birth would not be possible, the Consultant was off sick, and no one thought that he would agree to it anyway.

At 30 weeks I was told about another hospital 30 miles away, where a water birth had recently taken place. I wrote to the Director of Midwifery there, asking about the possibility of transferring there in order to have the birth we wanted. We were delighted to receive an almost instant reply saying that so long as there were no complications everything would be done to make our wish possible.

I next visited the hospital where I was originally booked at 32 weeks, to find the Consultant had returned to work and was not pleased that the senior midwives had held a meeting and decided against our having a water birth without consulting him about it.

ANNETTE
GASKELL

He said that we could have any birth we liked, and that he would see what he could do to arrange it with the hospital management, and would have a definite yes or no at my next visit at 34 weeks. Unfortunately, the answer was no, due to the Engineers Department being unhappy about whether the floor of the delivery suite would support the weight of the pool.

I went back to my GP then who arranged for the delivery to be booked at the second hospital. However, all was still not plain sailing as the letter went astray, and wasn't received until three weeks later, which meant that three weeks before the baby was due to arrive, we were still not booked in anywhere. Eventually, I telephoned the antenatal clinic myself and an appointment was made for me the following day.

From then on all went well. I took our pool to the hospital at my booking appointment and set it up in the delivery suite after booking in. I was shown round the delivery ward and made to feel welcome, and not at all that I was someone with an odd idea who would go away eventually. The midwives were enthusiastic and interested, and all wanted to know more about water births. I also saw the Director of Midwifery to whom I had written, and she confirmed again that if all went normally then our water birth would be supported, and my birth plan followed as far as possible. The Consultant too was happy for us to use the pool. The only matter of concern was that this was our third baby, and we lived so far from the hospital there might be problems travelling in labour, especially if we had to travel during the rush hour.

Over the next three weeks all was well, and there were no problems foreseen. I got to know several of the midwives and the one who had booked me in had been transferred to the labour ward. A midwife tutor had arranged to be present when we came into hospital, and there were instructions to contact her whatever the time.

My due date came and went. I now had appointments twice weekly. Ten days after my due date I began to have pains low down in my pelvis. Through the day the pains became stronger and more frequent. My sister took the children home with her. In the evening I telephoned Dave at work to say that I thought I was in labour and he came home at about 7 o'clock. At about 8 o'clock the pains stopped. Eventually, we went to bed, thinking that at least we could get a good night's sleep. I was glad that I hadn't called the hospital. About 2.00am I was awakened by another pain. I got pains then at irregular intervals for the rest of the night, about one or two an hour. In the morning we had an unexpected lie-in and got up at half past eight. I had a bath while

Dave made us some breakfast, and had three contractions in 10 minutes. After that the pains came more regular and frequent and we called the hospital, who told us to come in straight away. I hoped the traffic wouldn't be too heavy on the motorway, and I wouldn't have to deliver the baby on the hard shoulder. We arrived safely at the hospital at 11.30am and were met by the midwife tutor in the reception area. She took us up to the delivery suite where we were introduced to another midwife training to be a tutor. She took my blood pressure, pulse, etc., and listened to the baby's heartbeat using an ear trumpet. I had asked not to be monitored unless there were problems. She also felt the strength of my contractions manually and then examined me. I was four centimetres dilated.

The pool was filling and ready for me to get into at any time. I was pleased that the midwives took time to involve Dave in everything, and they explained all that was happening, and also that they took notice of our birth plan, and kept to our wishes. It's easy for people to agree with you in the antenatal clinic but it can be totally different when you arrive in labour.

Later, the midwife who had booked me in arrived on duty, and the tutors went for lunch. There was a leaving party going on for one of the midwives taking maternity leave, so the midwife brought some food for Dave so he wouldn't have to leave me while he went to get some lunch. I couldn't have anything to eat so I just had to watch between contractions while he tucked in.

I was still cheerful at this stage, breathing through the contractions, and managed to stay relaxed and walk about between contractions. The midwife brought a portable monitor so that we could hear the baby's heartbeat as she listened to it. Dave had listened through the pinnard, but obviously, I couldn't do that, so the sonicaid was a thoughtful gesture. As the contractions grew more painful, I decided I would get into the pool. We had been in hospital for about three hours by then.

I found the warm water helped a lot. I felt weightless, I could move easily and there was plenty of room to float about. At first the pains eased a great deal, but as I relaxed, the contractions soon became stronger and more painful. I thought I would get out for a while and stood up. Then I had another contraction and noticed the difference the water made to the level of pain, so I stayed in the pool.

At a quarter past four I was examined again. I was disappointed to learn that I was still only five centimetres dilated and thought that we might be there all night, although I knew that being relaxed in the water was supposed to help things speed up.

After another half an hour or so the contractions had become extremely painful and the midwife brought me gas and air which I had through a mouthpiece, not a mask, as she said the mask had a stronger effect and I could always change to that later on if necessary. I felt sick as well, so soon decided to get out of the water for a while, thinking I had plenty of time to get back in later.

I walked about for a while and tried sitting on the beanbag and on a chair, but the only place I felt comfortable was on a commode in a small adjoining room, hugging my gas and air. I had some backache by now as well as contractions and Dave helped a lot then by pulling on a towel around my hips which eased my backache but couldn't have done much for his arms.

I got back into the water for a while, and then out again. I found it difficult to get in as I could barely lift my leg by then, but getting out was easy as the water supported me. I sat back on the commode, still clinging on to my gas and air, although by this time I was biting so hard on the mouthpiece during each contraction that there couldn't have been much gas coming through.

At 5.35pm my waters broke. I was still sitting on the commode, so there was no flood of water on the floor. Almost immediately, I felt the urge to push so I got up. I would have liked to get back into the water but I couldn't lift my legs at all. It was all I could do to shuffle across to the bed. The midwife placed some steps beside the bed but I still couldn't get onto it. I couldn't move at all, I was frozen to the spot, and the baby was coming. Two more midwives arrived to assist, one of whom I had met before. Ten minutes later at 5.45pm, Helena was born, our third daughter, weighing 8lbs. The midwife said she had never delivered anyone standing up before. I found the birth itself easier than the first two, probably because gravity took over, and I didn't have to make much effort to push the baby out; she practically fell out.

Dave cut the cord, and counted her fingers and toes, then we waited for the placenta. I was still standing by the delivery bed and the midwives all went to get something to catch it in. As they came back, one behind me and one each side, the placenta dropped to the floor and nobody caught it which made us all laugh.

Somehow, I managed then to get onto the bed and I was relieved to find that I didn't need any stitches. After having a wash and the baby checked over, we were taken to the post-natal ward, where we stayed overnight and were discharged the following day.

Looking back, I felt more comfortable being in the care of a midwife I knew and it helped to know that nothing would be done that we didn't really want. There was no pressure put on us to conform to hospital policies, even though some of the things I had asked for were not standard procedure – for instance, I had asked not to be given Syntometrine during the third stage, on the assumption that if all was well and my uterus had been contracting well during first and second stage labour, there was no reason why it shouldn't continue to do so without help. Also, the use of the birthing pool was actively encouraged; people went out of their way to help in that respect.

In retrospect, I would have entered the water sooner if I had realised how it would speed things up and I would probably have stayed in for the delivery. The reason I got out was because I expected to have such a long time to go, yet only one and a half hours after being five centimetres dilated, our baby was born. The water did help a lot and I would definitely use the pool again if I had another baby.

An abbreviated version of this report appeared in Mother and Baby *magazine.*

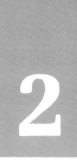

INDUCED AND ACCELERATED LABOURS

Sometimes pregnancy continues to 42+ weeks and induction is suggested. Other labours may start on time but need accelerating as they slow down. Our reports here range from a prostin gel induction onto the powerful contractions encouraged by a drip in accelerated labour. Although some women do not happily anticipate induction and are fearful of intervention, we have some reports where in fact it was welcome after a long pregnancy, and one where starting a first labour in the controlled hospital environment was very reassuring to the mother.

In retrospect I over-prepared myself for the experience of labour and childbirth. I manically read and re-read any relevant guidebooks, hospital literature and magazines I could lay my hands on and would loiter in libraries and bookshops trying to be able to envisage and experience my imminent ordeal. I had my hospital bags packed, just in case, when I was in my 30th week of pregnancy. Frequently, I lay awake at night timing the intervals between Braxton hicks contractions, worrying that labour would take me by surprise.

In the event, my son Joseph showed no such interest in the birthing experience and his arrival was eventually induced 10 days after his due date. Although the induction of birth sounded somewhat unnatural to me, it was actually very reassuring to have everything going on in the controlled atmosphere of the hospital. At 11 o'clock in the evening, prostin gel was applied to my cervix. Almost immediately, my waters broke and contractions began. The labour that followed took 17 hours and was 'normal' – that is as normal as such an intensely personal and unique experience as childbirth can be.

The least painful period of labour lasted from 11 o'clock at night to 9 o'clock the following morning. I also remember this period of labour as being the worst though, as I felt deeply isolated and lonely as I was not allowed to have my partner with me. Also, as I was spending the night on a full hospital ward which was ridiculously understaffed, the duty sister kept telling me to return to my bed and go to sleep, whilst all I wanted to do was walk around, moan a bit, and visit the loo to peer at my blood loss and escaping waters.

I felt relieved, emotional and crabby when my partner arrived in the morning. For three hours, we paced the wards, my partner patiently rubbing my back and doing controlled breathing with me as each contraction came. As the contractions got more frequent I found it easier to give way to the pain a bit – moan, sigh and feel sorry for myself. All that stuff I'd read about 'going' with each contraction seemed ridiculous, as I simply could not envisage a contraction increasing, reaching a plateau and dropping off. All I felt was pain.

As I entered the second stage of labour with the contractions becoming more frequent and intense, I asked for Pethidine, as I felt it was about time to have some help with the pain. The Pethidine was injected into my thigh and made me extremely nauseous. As the palaver of shifting me and my bags downstairs to the labour room took place around me, I fell asleep. For the next two hours I snatched fragments of sleep between

MIRANDA WALSH

contractions. As the contractions came more rapidly, I started inhaling Entonox. The mixture of Entonox and Pethidine made me extremely stoned and confused. At one point I believed I was on a chat show. My midwife who had a soft Irish accent became Terry Wogan. At another point I thought I was at a football match. The faces of the midwife, my partner and a trainee nanny who had requested to 'sit in' on the birth then merged into one and in my delirium I though I was stuck in a room with Wendy Craig. I remember (and have since been many times reminded by my partner) screaming 'action stations, evacuate Wendy Craig'.

Due to the large head of my baby, the second stage took quite some time. As the effects of Pethidine wore off, I became more level headed and the pain was excruciating. I felt as if someone was pulling a piece of wire, like a cheese cutter, through my insides. I kept reminding myself that it would be over soon, that this time tomorrow I would be somewhere else.

Finally, after a sudden rush and a dropping feeling, Joseph emerged. Looking down on the dazed new life, the duller pains of the afterbirth and the tear in my perineum were irrelevant. After all that effort and forever spent pregnant, here was a new person. After a quick hello and the separation of the umbilicus, Joseph was whisked away for a bit of oxygen. After an undignified rest with my legs stirruped up whilst my torn bits were sewn together, Joseph was returned bathed and sleepy. Rather than feeling tired I felt wildly awake with adrenalin and excitement.

See picture page 56

I know many ladies who consider childbirth a beautiful experience and with all sincerity I take my hat off to them. It is however with considerable regret that I must conclude that they either know something I don't, or that they possess an erogenous zone which I am lacking.

I gawp, open mouthed at tales I hear of pain-free natural labours, of water births, squatting, soft lights and music, and it is with real awe that I listen to those very clever (or very lucky) ladies who say 'I can't understand what all the fuss is about.'

I looked forward to the birth of our first child with some trepidation, but I think I was quietly confident that I could cope without too much ado.

Despite being rather too much on the portly side, I had during pregnancy, braved the aqua-natal classes, splashing and gasping away with the other mothers-to-be, all of them sylph-like apart from small neat 'bumps.' I heaved rather too many stones and a 'bump' which looked like it harboured a three year old around the pool smug in the knowledge that I was doing all I could to prepare myself for the forthcoming event.

At 38 weeks the big day came – or nearly came. A prostin induction of labour was arranged due to suspected placental insufficiency and we thought we would be parents before the day was done.

Two mothers-to-be, (myself included) were given prostin at 6.00am Saturday and examined four hours later. Mother-to-be number one was found to be three centimetres dilated and I waved her off to delivery with a flourish of the arms.

I was examined and told I hadn't budged a millimetre so the uncomfortable procedure was repeated. (This involves placing prostin gel beside the cervix) Another four hours passed. Mild contractions came and went. I breathed my way calmly through them. 'This' I thought, 'was going to be a doddle.'

The next examination revealed no progression and I was left to sleep on it. Sleep? That was a joke. Disheartened and miserable I fretted all night and got nary a wink – natch!

On Sunday, the by now familiar procedure was repeated twice more, the second attempt bringing such pain I thought I would lose my reason. Contractions came thick and fast and my screams could be heard reverberating around the maternity unit, frightening visitors and patients alike. Pethidine was offered and gratefully accepted (I hadn't even got to delivery yet) but by 3.00pm I was declared to be a lordly and impressive three centimetres dilated.

I was wheeled to delivery by a puffing midwife, the wheelchair tyres squeaking in protest and I hung my head in shame as we passed people whispering, 'Is that the screamer?'

Introductory pleasantries with my new midwife were cut short by my request for an epidural – something I had vowed not to have. Thank goodness I did. Many hours later, in foetal distress, Lydia was delivered with the assistance of forceps and an over-enthusiastic episiotomy, my legs were in stirrups, the lights blazed, my 'tail-end' faced the door, and half the town's population were in the room.

The whole experience from the beginning of induction to delivery had been a mere 42 hours and 5 minutes. Nevertheless I was desperately grateful to have a live, healthy baby. Weighing 6lb 12oz, we thought her utterly beautiful and my disappointment at such an awful experience was lost in my happiness and contentment in my little girl.

Two years later saw me approaching the birth of our second child. Friends reassured me that the second time around it was much easier, and my determination for a natural and hopefully beautiful birth intensified.

I practised squatting, rocking and breathing exercises, watched childbirth videos and asked countless questions. I had had over two years to prepare and this time I was going to get it right.

Again I had a prostin induced labour, this time only two days early. I received prostin at 8.00am and 12 midday and down to delivery I went. To cut a long story short, I screamed, I wailed, I begged, I pleaded, I shouted for the police, my solicitor, my mother – indeed anyone who, (in my Pethidine and Entonox affected state) may I thought be able to take away a pain which no-one deserved.

Eleanor, at 9lb 6oz, was born at 1.09am amidst blood, sweat, screaming, swearing, cursing and oceans of tears.

I loved her passionately on sight.

My experience of 'labour' resembles little the process described in the literature on the subject. Arriving at due date plus 15 days, it was decided that I should be admitted to the maternity wing serving an island community of 70,000 where there is an average of two births a day. The threat of being admitted for induction did nothing to spur my body on.

Due date plus 16 days, 10.00am – Young senior houseman (lady) appeared with syringe and 'dynogel' as it was nicknamed. I was soon to find out why. It was supposed to 'ripen' the cervix.

By lunchtime, I was having a few crampy feelings, but nothing more severe than I had experienced over the previous few weeks. My antenatal room mates spent the day giving me vivid descriptions of the sudden and dramatic effects that they had witnessed on the two ladies previously occupying my bed, who had had similar treatment.

The cheese salad predictably arrived at 4.30pm. This was the only vegetarian alternative to spam and chips. I was too uncomfortable to eat, anyway. There had been no measurable onset of labour, no definite contractions, and nothing that I was able to time. I was assured by a well meaning nurse that I couldn't be in labour, because I was still smiling. I called it a grimace!

My husband arrived at about 7.00pm and I moved into the labour room. The TENS apparatus had been fitted, but it was a disaster. Bob (my husband) who was operating it did not react nearly quickly enough to my orders, and I became frustrated and annoyed with him. So, after spending an hour leaning on a pillow over my bed head, it was into the bath. I am informed that contractions were now coming every 10 minutes. I seemed to have a constant pain around my abdomen (the baby was facing forwards and not engaged). Lying back in the bath gave no relief, indeed, if anything it made things worse – I wanted to lean forwards. This also facilitated me being sick at regular intervals, although there was nothing left to throw up by now.

I was heaved out of the bath shortly after 9.00pm, but the contractions were so violent and frequent that there was no time to get dry. I started to shake and this didn't stop until well after the baby was born.

The next three hours were sheer hell. No brave active labour for me, as I had so meticulously planned. I was just a writhing lump on the bed. The pain was constant, back and front. It felt as though I was in the grip of a vice, but inside-out. The room was dark, Julian Lloyd-Webber was soothingly bowing on his cello strings, but to no effect. During the slight and brief respite which I did get, I seem to remember my eyes rolling up into my head, as

SUSAN PYNEGAR

I sank into a semi-conscious state. I began to dread the next excruciating pain. I think I opened my eyes twice during the period up to midnight. The first time, I saw Bob asleep bolt upright! The second time I was disturbed by a strange noise. He was crunching raw carrots! These had been intended for me, had I been bored!

Shortly after 10.00pm the midwife decided that she should examine me to see how far dilated I was. I was aghast at the news it was only three centimetres. I could not believe that the pain could get more severe.

By about 11.45pm, I was absolutely at the end of my tether, and against all my strongly held principles, I was asking for anything which could relieve me. Pethidine was the only thing available here. (Epidurals had to be booked well in advance). The midwife, on consultation with my husband, was reluctant to administer any, as she knew how I felt about such matters. I remember asking, 'How long is this going to go on? I can't go on like this till morning.' The consensus was to wait another 30 minutes. She was apparently becoming quite concerned.

12.45am came and went, and she decided that I had had enough. Although she wasn't very confident that internally much progress had been made, she did make a check – eight and a half centimetres! Action stations were called. Gas and air was wheeled in. I don't know whether it had any pain relieving qualities, but at least I had something to concentrate on, and I thought we had moved into the delivery room. I heard my husband ask if the gas and air was a hallucinogen. I shouted, 'I'm not mad, you know. Ha Ha. I've still got my sense of humour!'

12.40am approximately. I began to feel the need to push, but was told to wait. 12.50am, my waters broke. They were meconium stained. A doctor was called. I was told to start pushing very hard, because unless the baby was born quickly he was going to be very sick. The pushing process took 12 minutes – it was the easiest part, apart from when his head came out (facing the correct way). I felt as though I were being operated on without anaesthetic! Only a slight tear though, and no episiotomy!

Edwin was born at 1.07am on the 20th of February 1991. He was laid on my tummy but the cord had to be cut quickly as he needed resuscitation. Apgar scores four and six. He was a long, slithery little being and looked most concerned. After 36 hours in special care, he thrived and is now a beautiful specimen.

See picture page 55

At around my 36th week of pregnancy, it was decided that I may have to have a Caesarean section as my baby was breech. I had a pelvic X-Ray and this showed that there was enough room for the baby to be born. On my antenatal visit during week 40, it was decided that I would be induced. They seemed to have it all organised. As this is my only child, I didn't know what to expect.

I was only allowed to go nine days overdue. On 31st October, I had my last antenatal visit and went straight up to the labour ward. At 6 o'clock the next day, I went down to the delivery suite to wait for the doctor. A nurse came and put a glucose and saline drip into my wrist. It was the most horrible thing that anyone has ever done to me! I was given a tablet and a thimble sized cup of water to dry up the fluids in my stomach just in case I had to have an emergency Caesarean. I had also had one of the tablets at 11 o'clock the previous night. I was really thirsty! I waited in the room for three more hours until the doctor arrived. She was familiar to me as she had done a few of my antenatal checks. She examined me and said that it would be best if I was prepared for a Caesarean birth as the baby's feet were presenting first, but were pressing down as well. I had been two centimetres dilated for about two weeks already. She asked for a second opinion though and another doctor said that in view of the pelvic x-ray that I had had, it would be much better to have a trial of labour and see how things progressed. At 10 o'clock the doctor inserted a pessary into my vagina. Me and my drip went into a sitting room to see how things went. My husband and mum had been with me since about 8 o'clock which was really great. At 12.30pm I had had only one contraction! So they decided to break my waters and set up another drip to speed up the labour.

They broke my waters and it felt as if I had been sick through the other end. It was hot and sloppy. I was soaked! But even though it hurt, I could cope. That was until the drip was turned on. In one contraction the pain went from quite strong to breathtaking. I couldn't breathe. I had been to all the parentcraft classes and I had learnt the breathing techniques but it didn't seem to work. I just burst into tears! The midwife was wonderful. She really helped me to relax and kept telling me that my contractions were only so powerful because the drip had to be on high. My baby had to be born as quickly as possible as it was important that she didn't get stuck. I had agreed to have an epidural if I did need a Caesarean, so I could be awake.

After about half an hour, the midwife asked me if I wanted it. I said no at first (trying to be brave) but soon gave in. The

JOSEPHINE DOWD

anaesthetist's junior did my epidural. I didn't feel anything. I was put down on my back again and told that in a few minutes I would not feel anything. The monitor that I had strapped to my bump was really digging in. The bedding had still not been changed since my waters were broke. I felt scared and wet! A few minutes later the anaesthetist came in and asked me how I felt. It hadn't worked and I felt horrible. He topped up the epidural and said he'd be back soon. He came back and it still hadn't worked. He removed the tube fom my back. Tearing off the strip of plaster that held it down was very painful. The junior had put the tube in too high up in my spine which explained why my hands and mouth were numb! He did it again. This time it hurt because I could not relax. My contractions were lasting two and three minutes and were only seconds apart. Once again I was put on my back – and once again it didn't work! So he topped it up again. This time, one leg and the side of my hips went totally dead. My right leg went dark red and very hot. By this time my mum and husband were getting really tired. I think my husband felt useless. He looked sorry for me! The pain on one side was so bad; however, I still fell asleep for an hour and a half!

When I woke up it was 6.30ish. The epidural had virtually worn off on my other hip. My leg was still totally numb. A midwife came in and sat me up. The bedding still hadn't been changed but my bum was a bit dead so I couldn't feel it. At 7 o'clock I got a pain in my back. I remember saying to my mum and husband 'I think this is it.' I pressed the midwife's bell and she came in. I explained about the back pain. The doctor was called for and she examined me. 'Push on the next contraction.' YES!! At last! I couldn't tell my contractions apart though because the pain had washed over me. I pushed. I felt quite daft though because I thought my eyes would pop out. The doctor examined me again. Amy's right leg had come down but her left leg was stuck up her back. She was also facing the wrong way and her arms were folded under her chin. The doctor put both hands in to feel. Then she said, 'push as if you're going to the loo.' Well, I did and I poohed! I felt awful! In front of my husband and my mum! Not only that, but Amy did it too.

Next thing my legs went in stirrups. This was about 7.45pm. By this time two midwives, husband, mum, anaesthetist, junior, doctor and paediatrician were with me. The doctor did an episiotomy, put both hands in and turned Amy round. I sat up to push about twice more and Amy was born at 7.49pm weighing 7lb 15oz. I cried my eyes out! All I wanted to know was whether or not she was alive!

I was stitched and my legs taken out of stirrups. The bedding was the original bedding that was on when my waters were broken and because of this I gained two blisters as big as small eggs at the base of my spine. They were caused by friction of my sitting forward to push. Two hours later the drips were taken out. I was washed and sent up to the post-natal ward.

The first hour or so after birth, I just gazed at Amy and my husband cuddled me. It was the best moment ever. I just couldn't believe that this wonderful person came out of me! I breastfed her and loved it. After I had been home a few weeks I realised what I had gone through. I couldn't imagine why anyone would have themselves put through that more than once. I was over that feeling soon though.

Although I will feel quite scared of labour when I face it again, and although I'll never erase that day from my mind, I'll always look back on it with pride. I'll never get over doing the poohs though! I really can't wait for baby number two now because it's worth it. The pain is lost when the baby is in your arms.

See picture page 127

3

ASSISTED DELIVERIES – FORCEPS, VENTOUSE AND CAESAREAN

Deliveries do not always fit our birth plans and some babies need assistance in the form of forceps, ventouse extraction or Caesarean section. Sometimes, we hear that women feel they have failed if they need assistance to deliver their babies, or feel negative towards their children. We hope that the reports here show that assisted deliveries can be positive, and are not as fearful as many women imagine; they do not always repeat themselves and do not have to interfere with the mother/baby bond or inhibit breastfeeding. Caesareans range from elective, using epidural, or spinal anaesthesia to emergency situations using general anaesthesia.

June 7th, 1988, 39 weeks plus three days. A 12 hour labour. 8.30am. After two weeks experiencing Braxton Hicks I knew that the 'gripping' pains meant something different. I told my husband the baby would probably come today as he went off to work.

9.00am. Did washing and shopping. Carried the lot home in a pack on my back – definitely having contractions.

12.00am. Light lunch, went to loo and had slight show, no blood (hadn't expected it to be clear).

12.30am. After speaking to my husband Michael (a doctor) he convinced me to pack my bags in preparation. I was visiting hospital for my antenatal tour. I had always been concerned about getting there from home (I had suggested the bus!) and so I now had the opportunity of a lift and I could be monitored to see if it was 'for real.' Contractions, very mild, were coming at between five and ten minutes.

1.30pm. Friend arrived to see me bags in hand. She drove slowly down the hill to avoid my waters breaking! Contractions every five minutes.

2.00pm. Did our tour – contractions all the while but mild.

2.30pm. Told a midwife I thought I was in labour. Organised monitoring. Friend sat with me during ¾ hour – could see my contractions coming up and wondered why I wasn't in pain. Had complete show – contractions still five minute intervals but irregular strength.

4.00pm. Friend and I laughed as she left – my flying visit was to become an overnight stay! Gave her a few numbers to ring 'in case.'

4.30pm. Female doctor told me it was probably a false alarm, but she wanted to admit me because my blood pressure was up! Contractions still every five minutes. Depressed me in case it was all for nothing.

5.15pm. Michael arrived to chat and to try and cheer me up. He'd always said the baby would be born on June 7th. He was close.

5.45pm. Light supper so Michael went to get some nourishment himself – the only thing not packed in my rush! Contractions still every five minutes.

6.30pm. Michael returned and we went walking as contractions continued. Stronger now and more regular at five minute intervals. A beautiful evening for a stroll. Found fossils in the hospital car park!

7.55pm. Sat on a brick wall and my waters broke! Amazed how much there was. Very amusing as we negotiated the hospital

ANN YOUNG

corridors with me dripping more at each contraction.

8.15pm. Contractions every four minutes and very intense. Not coping well. Trying to use antenatal relaxation but strength of contractions overwhelming. Watched the puddle of water grow on the floor by the bed as each contraction forced more fluid out. Clutching the radiator greatly helped.

8.20pm. The woman opposite me in antenatal ward told by doctor she had lost a 42-week baby. In pain and out of control I felt very vulnerable for the safety of mine.

8.30pm. Moved to labour ward. Tried rocking chair, walking, leaning on bed. Contractions so intense, nothing helped. Still every five minutes. Vivaldi Four Seasons on the tape was distracting.

9.30pm. Gas and air, but couldn't get co-ordinated. Kept thinking I was missing the contractions!

10.00pm. Pethidine seemed the answer to coping. Watched the sunset. Realised I was totally stoned! I remember saying I thought childbirth was worth it for the drugs.

10.15pm. Consultant (it sometimes helps to be a doctor's wife) and admitting doctor visited. Joked with them about my false labour.

10.20pm. Examined by midwife – only four centimetres dilated.

11.00pm. Still four centimetres dilated and contractions still ferocious. Pethidine affected Baby's heart rate – very low. Scalp monitor for baby.

June 8th, 12.30am. Pethidine wearing off – Pain and still four centimetres dilated. Decided to have an epidural. (In fact, Michael helped; I was too out of control to know what to do!).

1.00am. Drip set up (Glucose).

1.30am. Epidural administered.

1.40am. Feeling first effects – wonderful release from pain and able to nap. Baby's heart rate excellent.

2.15pm. Beginning to wear off – feeling contractions in left side.

2.30am. Topped up.

4.00am. Fully dilated! The last few hours had been very hazy as I was weary from my earlier exertions.

5.30pm. After the epidural had worn off, I began to push with each contraction, but it was no good. The baby kept slipping back. Felt very weary and pushing was hard work as I had no urge.

6.20am. Consultant arrived to help the baby out. Epidural

topped up again.

6.35am. Organised me for a forceps delivery. People everywhere, but by then I didn't care – I just wanted my baby born. Scalp monitor removed – very quiet without her bips and a little disconcerting.

6.45am. Pushed with each contraction. I could feel the progress of the baby down as pressure, but no pain.

6.57am. Baby Madeleine appeared with a final effort. She looked a little blue but her lungs told the real story!

7.00am. I had our baby in my arms, as the placenta was delivered. She went easily to the breast.

7.15am. Stitched up, but oblivious to most of the goings-on as I held our baby close. At 8lb 2¹/₂ oz, she wasn't a bad specimen.

7.30am. All the attendents had left as we became a family. We were left alone until 8.00pm – I slept for most of that, after losing my first welcome cup of tea!

8.00am. Moved to small room to have my blood pressure monitored as it was high. Felt very tired, but incredibly pleased with myself, despite all the intervention. Michael went off to spread the good news and take the morning off work.

Afterthoughts:
Both Michael and I were really impressed with the care at hospital. No one ever forced us to make a decision – they suggested what they thought was best, but would have been supportive had I wished the birth to have been different. I was disappointed things hadn't gone more naturally, but I was pleased that baby Madeleine was perfect and that more than compensated.

A second labour – Ann Young, now in Australia
At 36 weeks I had a false labour, so I expected our new arrival any day and re-read my labour report of three years previous to 'refresh' my memory. I was expecting a six or seven hour labour – about 'right' I thought.

At 9.00am on 10th December my waters broke while watering the garden.

9.14am. Rang husband to come home, telling him not to rush; arranged for a neighbour to take my three year old and watered my indoor plants.

9.30am. Rang hospital and had my first contraction. Midwife told me not to rush!

10.00am. Contractions three minutes and regular. Husband home, and then back to hospital across city traffic. Not too uncomfortable.

10.30am. Admitted to labour ward with strong contractions two minutes apart. Only three centimetres dilated, but cervix thin! At this stage I needed some gas and air and felt I might have a long day ahead of me and perhaps a repeat performance of labour number one.

10.35am. Felt sick, contractions strong. Looked out of window across harbour, and I remember seeing some yachts in full sail. I contemplated ever so briefly that it was a great day and place to be born!

11.00am (I think). Contractions very strong and fast. Midwives left us to it and contacted our obstetrician who was coming in at 1.30pm to see me. At this stage I felt out of control. The contractions were very strong and coming on top of each other. I remember lying on the delivery bed, thinking I would have to have another epidural if this keeps up.

11.15am. Felt an odd pressure in my belly and apparently grunted. Michael asked me if I needed to push and I replied, 'Yes'. What a relief. He looked down to see baby crowning and called for a midwife.

Next five minutes I remember grunting, pushing, straining and stretching. After three or four pushes our baby boy was born at 11.29am! I was in shock, it was so quick. I couldn't believe a baby could come so quickly. My obstetrician arrived just as Michael cut the cord. the doctor was also surprised at the rapid birth. The baby did not feed immediately but yelled a little. His father took him while the resultant tear was stitched up after the placenta was delivered.

A speedy birth indeed – an 8lb 9oz baby boy born in just two hours, and just one hour from three centimetres to delivery! My body and mind were in shock – that afternoon, some three hours later, it dawned on me I had another baby (Jeremy). I could have gone out and danced I felt so good.

See picture page 128

This was my first pregnancy, which was completely planned and both myself and my husband were absolutely delighted. Right from the start I was determined that I wanted the birth itself to be as natural as possible, and initially looked into giving birth at home. After taking on the local family practitioner committee, midwives, etc., and having to change GP, we reached a compromise that I would be booked into a GP unit at a local maternity hospital, delivered by one of the team of local community midwives and return home within eight hours of the delivery – providing that the rest of my pregnancy proved normal.

I was therefore absolutely horrified when towards the end of my pregnancy the baby refused to turn round as my GP (who was supposed to deliver the baby) said, 'I'm afraid this is where we part company – good luck!'

On Friday 6th September, I was sent to the hospital antenatal department for final scan and pelvic x-rays to determine the next course of action to take. After waiting hours in various departments, I finally got to see the lady Registrar who looked at all the results and said that I would have to have a Caesarean, asked whether I would prefer general or spinal anaesthetic and after checking her diary said, 'come to the ward on Monday at 1.00pm – see you in theatre on Tuesday.' I was at this stage 37$^{1}/_{2}$ weeks pregnant.

I left the hospital in somewhat of a daze, having been given virtually no information, no leaflets and nothing verbal to let me know what to expect at all. Whereupon when I got home I tried to calmly tell my husband that he would be a father on Tuesday.

That was the strangest thing of all – knowing in advance D-Day was Tuesday 10th September. I didn't know whether to tell people or not – somehow I felt embarrassed, I don't know why; also, it destroyed all my feelings of anticipation. I wanted to surprise people not tell them in advance – the only thing to look forward to was not knowing the baby's sex. In the end we agreed to inform close family only in advance and leave friends until later.

I hadn't finished preparations at all and up until only a few hours ago I had still been hoping for a natural delivery and not to have to stay in hospital absolutely longer than necessary. At least such short notice was good in some ways – I didn't have time to brood too much, although after having a telephone conversation with my mother regarding her hysterectomy and a similar one with my sister in law regarding her two Caesareans. I had some more idea of what to expect and madly rushed out to buy extra nighties, waist high 'granny' briefs, etc, extra disposables for the long stay in hospital as nothing at all was provided due to cut-

JANET
CULLINGFORD

backs. I didn't sleep too well Sunday night. Paul left for work as usual; he was meeting me at the hospital later to settle me in. I must have been worried as I solemnly wrote him a letter in case I didn't survive the experience and left it under his pillow. I met Paul at 1.00pm in the foyer of the maternity department, so we went up together. I was given a private room with TV just for the night before the big day (so that I wasn't disturbed by crying babies).

I felt completely isolated and ignored – all alone in my little room – after Paul had gone. A nurse came in and shaved me and left me on a foetal monitor for a while. Around 7.00pm the Consultant came round to check me over – didn't say very much and certainly didn't invite my confidence – it then became apparent that not only had I been ignored, they'd even forgotten to get me an evening meal – they were very apologetic and gave me some toast. When Paul came to visit I sent him out for fish and chips.

Around 11.00pm the anaesthetist came to visit, another lady who quite frankly terrified me – she gave verbal descriptions of the whole procedure ending with, 'and if you can't bear the pain I'll give you gas and air or Pethidine – if it becomes too much I can always knock you out.' I was then petrified. I'd opted for a spinal block because I wanted to be awake but I thought that meant I wouldn't feel it at all. I found it very hard to sleep after her 'comforting' visit.

D-Day. Tuesday 10th September. I was awake just after 5.00am after a terrible night – very hungry and thirsty, nervous. My main fear at that point stupidly was that the porter would arrive to take me to the theatre before Paul did. Paul arrived at 9.00am as requested – he looked as white as I did. I got gowned up; a staff nurse came in and gave me a handful of tablets, then the trolley arrived. All the way to theatre Paul held my hand.

First stop he was taken away to get into operating robes, mask, etc., but the theatre staff (all female) were quite good and just chatted until he returned. First of all was the spinal; this was the worst part of all. I had to sit on the edge of a high trolley with my feet on a stool. They put a table in front of me and told me to lean on it with my arms crossed. They then sat Paul in front of me and asked him to pin my arms down.

I could feel the needle going in and in over and over again – it was agonising pain and took them 35 minutes to get it in the right place – apparently I was just very unlucky; also not helped by a spinal injury caused by a car accident a few years earlier. Eventually, they pronounced they were satisfied and lay me down

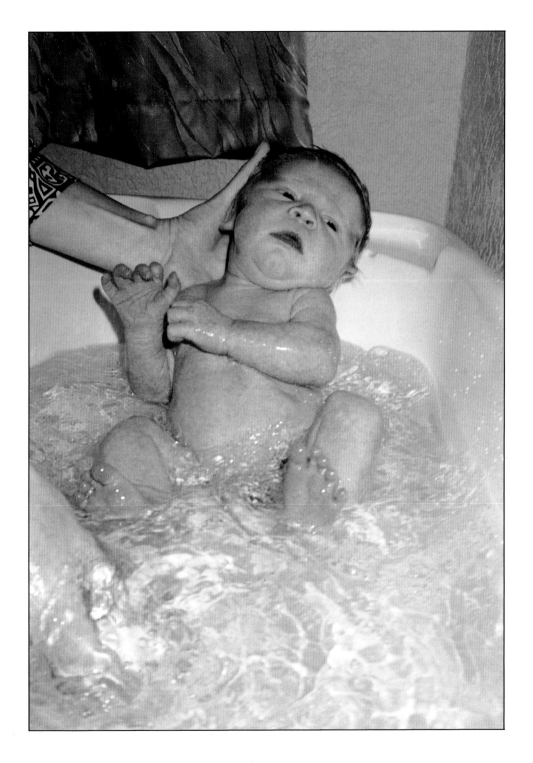

James Ormond age 1 month

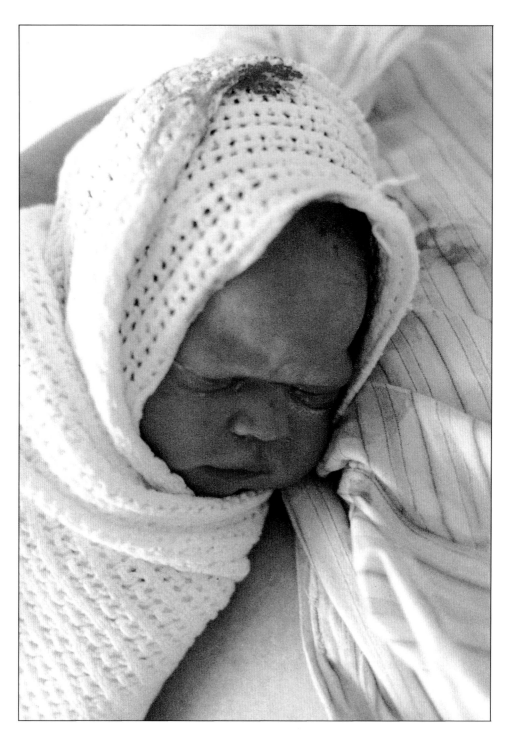

Ruth Eloise Lewis . . . just 5 minutes old

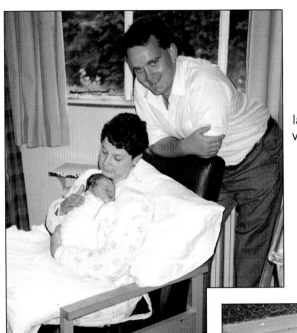

Ian and Jane Northcott
with Laura Jane (*left*)

2 day old Edwin Lindsay with
mum Susan Pynegar (*right*)

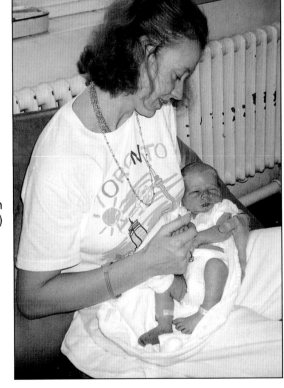

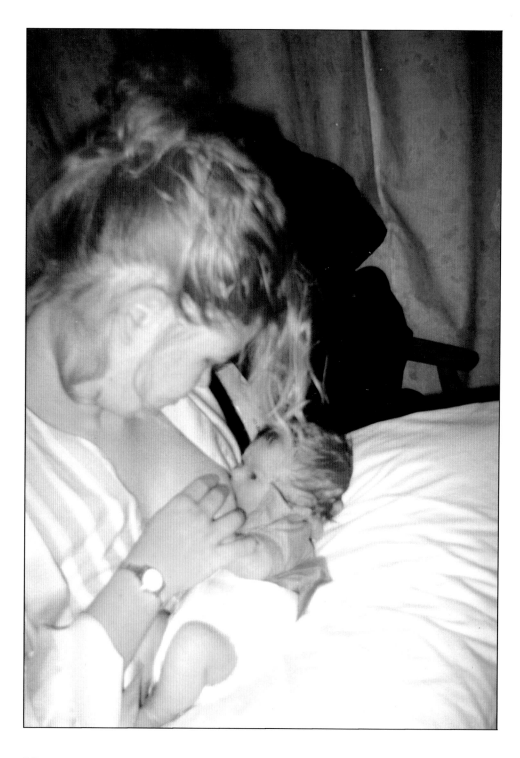

Miranda Walsh giving baby Joseph his first breast feed

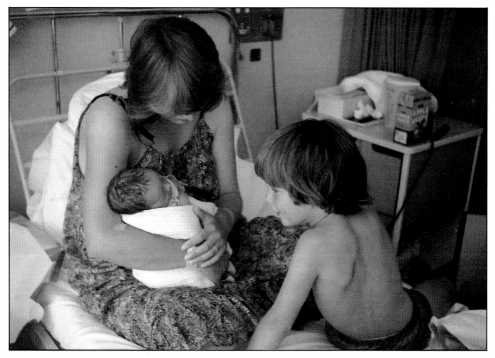

Judith Martin with Daniel and Rosamund (*above*)

Jo Stewart with Jamie and baby Camilla (*below*)

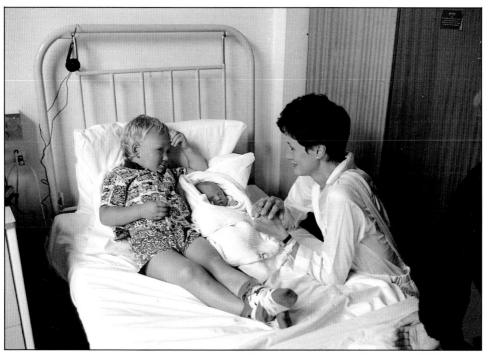

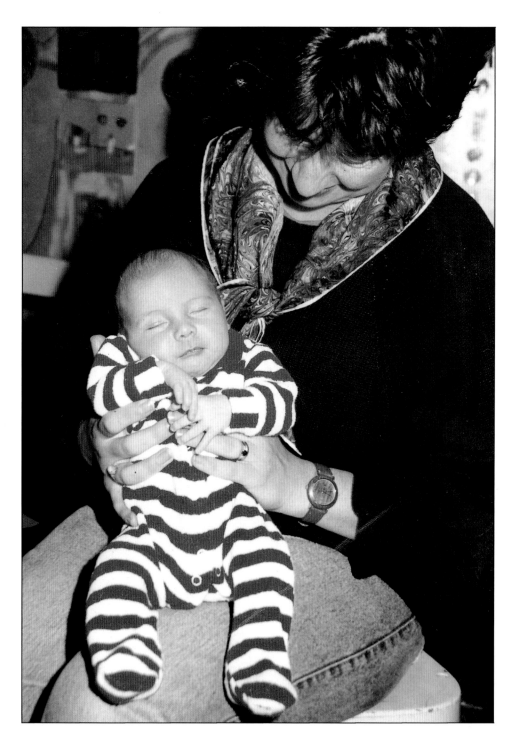

Christine Hogg and Joseph

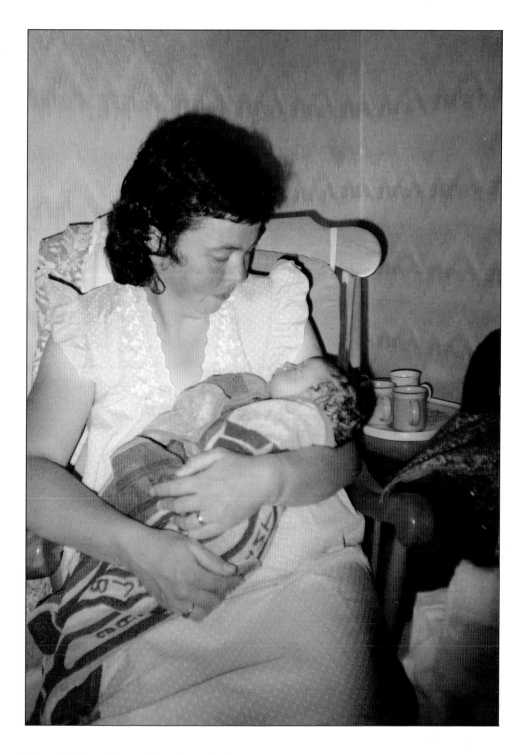

Karen Hibbs with son Gareth on dry land

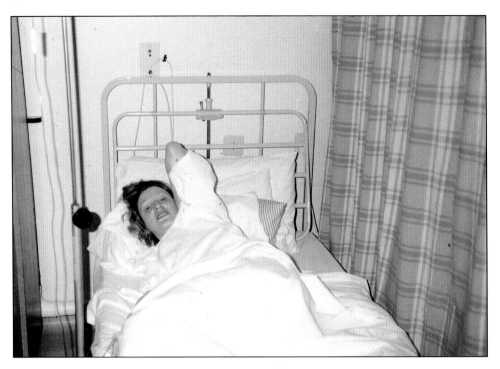

Dawn Robinson-Walsh recovering from general anaesthetic after giving birth . . .
and Alexandra Jennie sleeping it off

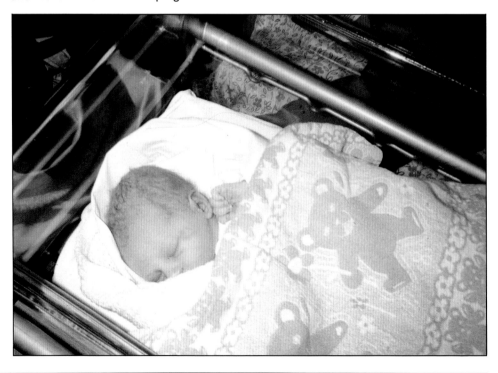

again. I lay there for a few minutes while they inserted a drip and they kept looking at my blood pressure, then sprayed ice cold stuff on my stomach and kept doing that until I couldn't feel it and then tested again with a needle – then into the theatre itself I was wheeled. I must confess once I actually got into the anaesthetic room the staff were very good, friendly and constantly explaining what they were doing and why they were doing it, but my mind was completely closed to most of it; that part mostly is now a blank.

I was next lifted onto the operating table – they found Paul a stool at my right hand shoulder and he sat down and held my hand – they put a screen up so that neither of us could see but I didn't look anyway. I just gazed fixedly into his eyes all the time.

I can honestly say that I felt no pain at all. I felt them cutting me open but it didn't hurt; it was a very strange feeling because I could feel their hands inside me moving around but I was detached from it altogether. I heard a sort of pump sucking out all the amniotic fluid then a tugging sensation. They shouted, 'look over to your left,' and I saw them carrying off a baby to a table in the corner. It didn't cry and momentarily I panicked, then I heard a cry and they said, 'it's a lovely little girl – what are you going to call her?' I looked at Paul who had tears streaming down his face – I can honestly say I didn't feel a thing emotionally, I just thought 'so what? It's a baby. I don't care!' I didn't feel any love, maternal instinct or anything. I was so detached. Paul said, 'Erin' which was the name we'd chosen, and we both watched the paediatricians dealing with her in the far corner, cleaning her up, etc . . . while they stitched me up. When they'd finished stitching they brought her over and put her in Paul's arms and I just looked at her. I couldn't believe how tiny she was (6lb 7oz), much dark hair and beautiful eyes – but they wouldn't let me hold her. I couldn't have done anyway as there was very little sensation in my arms.

She was then put in a perspex cot which Paul was given to wheel back to the ward. I was trolleyed back alongside.

It must have been around 11.00am as the stitching took a long time. Back on the ward I was pushed into a bay of four beds. They didn't pull the curtains round as I was the only one in that bay anyway which was reserved for Caesareans. Paul sat at my side and a nurse came up and sat on the other side to hold the baby to me to try her first feed. She sucked very well which surprised me. After a few minutes on each nipple, they gave her back to Paul to hold and left us alone staring at our baby. I still felt very few emotions. I thought she was pretty and so perfect in the way only a new baby is, but it was more of a detached observation. Paul was ecstatic. I had so many doubts but there was no turning back now; she was ours for life.

We sat there together for over an hour; no-one asked Paul to leave, they brought him tea and biscuits. Eventually, around 1.00pm, he decided to go home and ring all the family and return at afternoon visiting. I felt disappointed that I couldn't share such a pleasurable task with him and when he returned later I wanted to know every last word and nuances of expressions that people had used – I felt a little left out – and guilty that I wasn't as happy as they tell you you are supposed to be.

Unfortunately, by this time the spinal was wearing off and I was in agony – even to breathe hurt – injections took the edge off it – later I remember I was left there in so much pain, tears streaming silently down my face, biting my lips and gritting my teeth. The ward cleaning lady noticed and despite my protestations went to find a nurse who rather abruptly said I was only allowed one more injection and I would be better to save it until later to help me through the night and promptly offered me two paracetamol.

The sequence of events is not clear in my mind probably due to the pain and the drugs used, etc., but throughout the rest of the day, staff came round to take my temperature, BP, check stitches, etc., help me feed the baby, change her, etc. I couldn't move at all – every time she cried I had to ring the bell; I felt so useless. I didn't really feel she was mine at all. Certainly none of this maternal bonding bit. When Paul returned at evening visiting hours he sat with Erin in his arms next to me and just gazed at her in wonder. I felt it was the baby he wanted to see and not me at all.

The day after the delivery was the worst for me. I felt very ill and weak. I had lost any high at all that I had had about having Erin and was very down. I still had the drip in and the catheter and couldn't move at all. Then a nurse came to try and get me out of bed to help me have a shower. As soon as they got me out of bed I haemorrhaged very badly. I was really frightened with the blood, people running everywhere. They more or less threw me back on the bed and got a doctor.

No-one told me anything. I didn't know what was normal to feel or be like and began to wonder if something had gone wrong during the operation that I didn't know about. While I was in hospital another girl came in to have a Caesarean and afterwards she was much better than I had been. I got more depressed as the day went on. I had no visitors in the afternoon which was so depressing and then once evening visiting was over and Paul had gone I felt the lowest I have ever felt in my life. I began to cry and just couldn't stop; nothing any of the nurses said helped. They gave me sedatives. I just blubbered on and on. Eventually around 1 o'clock in the morning they rang Paul and got him to come out to the hospital and offer his comfort.

I hated my entire stay in hospital; some of the staff were very abrupt and uncaring; one or two were great, especially my little cleaning lady. I was hungry all the time as I wasn't allowed anything at all for two days and then only soup and ice cream for three days which demoralised me. Once I got out of bed I found walking very difficult and was nervous of picking up Erin, changing her, etc. I didn't fully relax until I got home. Worst of all once the catheter was removed I had terrible problems going to the toilet. I remember crying a lot over that. I have been told that it is probable that I will have to have another Caesarean if I have any more children but that hasn't put me off; in fact, we're trying for a baby right now. At least next time I'll know what to expect.

I didn't feel cheated in the end that I didn't have a natural delivery. I think that was because I knew in advance and had time to get over that aspect of it: it was more the physical aspects of it that I resented. It seemed like weeks before I could stand up straight, have a bath alone, even silly things like not being able to drive for six weeks took away my freedom.

Emotionally my main problem was that I didn't feel I loved the baby: that took a long time to come, months in fact. I felt this was unnatural and agonised about it for weeks. I didn't think that I could take to her at all. I actually had to force myself to communicate with her; it felt unnatural and wrong somehow. I could feed her and change her, bath her, but took no particular pleasure in it. I certainly didn't want to play with her.

Erin is now 10 months old and I have now come to realise that I am not the usual kind of mother or not the sort I imagined I would be. I love her dearly and wouldn't be without her for the world but I still find the day to day tasks easier to carry out than the supposedly enjoyable ones. Sometimes I still have to force myself to play with her and talk to her but I have begun to believe that that is just me and I'm by no means the only person like this. In some ways I think it is quite good for her — she is learning to be self-sufficient and can amuse herself for short periods of time. She has turned out to be a very placid, contented baby who does nothing but smile and laugh and gurgle all the time. All my friends with similar age babies are envious of her sweet nature. Wherever I go I get stopped by people telling me how beautiful she is and good natured. I'll probably get a shock with the next one.

PAT
AITCHISON

My first child, Kathy, was born by elective section. Although there had been talk of a possible section for some time – the baby was also said to be large and I am only five feet – it was still a bit of a shock to be told that a section would be performed the next day. By this time I was already 13 days overdue. The baby was large and lying obliquely, so really there was little alternative. Everything was fully and sympathetically explained both by the Consultant and the other staff. My husband, Iain, who was present at the antenatal session was also involved and part of the decision.

I had always dreaded deciding what sort of anaesthetic I would prefer in 'cold blood' but now I had to do so. Iain did not particularly fancy being present at a full operation and rather hoped that I would choose a general so that he could not be there. I was quite surprised when I heard my own voice asking for an epidural quite, I'm sure, of its own volition. The Consultant assured me that they could give me a general at any time if I really hated it and reassured Iain that he would see less blood than at a normal birth. All this happened at about 2.30pm on the Wednesday and I was then told to go home, relax, sort myself out and return for admission at 6–6.30pm that evening.

When I was admitted there was plenty of time for explanations, queries and generally finding out exactly what would happen. Iain came in with me and stayed until about 9.00pm (although official visiting finished at 8.00pm). He was at all times made welcome and encouraged to feel part of the whole event. When he left, he knew at what time he needed to be back in the morning and what would happen.

The next morning, after a bath and no breakfast, we were taken down to theatre where we met everyone who was to be involved. I was glad to find that the doctors performing the operation were two women whom I had met fairly often at antenatal visits. This provided a good feeling of continuity.

I found the setting up of the epidural fairly trying (particularly as I have always hated needles) but everyone was so pleasant and concerned that I was alright; it was not as bad as expected. The feeling of light-headedness that the anaesthetic produced was really strange but a whiff of oxygen helped enormously.

The operation itself was so quick that I could not believe it when the Doctor announced that we had a daughter. Iain had actually taken up the invitation to look over the green screen erected across my chest to see the baby born. He was relieved, I think, that all he could see was the baby coming out of a hole in a sheet, no blood or horrors. I hadn't felt a thing.

The subsequent part of the procedure I found not entirely painless. At one point I said, I am told, 'Bloody hell, that hurts!' and they gave me gas and air. I had been warned that I would feel some tugging and pulling but this did actually hurt. It turned out that it was the cleaning out process that caused the problem. I did in fact have a post partum haemorrhage, I later discovered.

As soon as Kathy had been weighed she was handed to Iain who held her next to me so that I could touch and stroke her although I could not hold her myself. Such are the effects of mixed anaesthesia and euphoria that Kathy was over two years old when I discovered that she screeched during most of this period. Once in the recovery room she was put to my breast where she found absolutely no joy at all. I never did produce any milk for her, poor thing.

I was confined to bed for the rest of that day but the next morning they got me up for a shower. I swear that the 40 yards or so to the bathroom were more like four miles that morning, although the distance decreased substantially every day. I found that recovery did not take nearly as long as I expected and quite amazed myself by walking down three flights of stairs only four days after Kathy was born.

All the staff were superb and I never felt under any pressure. I could have left hospital on the fifth day but they sensed my reluctance. They asked again on the sixth but on the seventh I knew myself to be ready and that is when I left. I never felt the sense of failure that so many women reputedly do because I had had a section, and was hugely relieved when advised, after pelvic x-rays were examined, that subsequent deliveries should be sections unless the baby was a real tiddler.

By the time my second baby was conceived, we had moved to Lancashire and I found the whole experience to be quite different. It was agreed this time round at 36 weeks that a section would be performed at 39 weeks gestation. I felt this time that although my views were taken into account eventually, that it was in spite of everyone's better judgement and that I was a little strange in pushing myself and my view forward. Husbands were not expected to attend antenatal sessions at the hospital although they were permitted a short glimpse of the scan. This was not explained at the time, as it had been before, but you were sent to antenatal just to be told, 'it's fine, dear.' Questions were, I felt, discouraged. This all left me feeling somewhat unhappy and unsure of myself and the situation.

I was told that I was to be admitted at no later than 2.30pm the day preceding the operation despite me asking if it could be later in order that I could spend that last afternoon at home with Kathy. In fact I saw no one nor underwent any preparatory procedures until well into the evening and spent the afternoon very much at a loose end. At the other hospital, visiting was 2–8pm and flexible outside that but here it was 2–3pm and 7–8pm and that was even for husbands. Iain felt very excluded, understandably. There was no clear idea of when Iain should return the next morning – one midwife suggested he telephone at 9.30am. In the end he came in at 8.30am and we went up to theatre at 9.45am. Luckily he did not take the advice to ring later on.

On this occasion I had been advised to have a spinal anaesthetic in preference to an epidural and I am glad that I took the advice. It was much easier and quicker to set up and took away all sensation from the relevant area. The drawback was that I felt much more light-headed throughout the whole procedure and seemed to need a lot of oxygen which was rather distracting. They also wrapped my arms close to my chest so that when Michael was born I was unable to touch him until the recovery room, when my arms were freed. Although slightly slower than previously – nine minutes from start to birth rather than four – the actual operation was again a wonderful experience. All the staff were very pleasant although I had met none of them before. I am sure that all anaesthetists must attend some sort of training in amusing patients who are awake! We seemed to spend the whole time laughing – it was wonderful.

I had decided from the start that Mike would be bottle fed as I did not know whether I would have any milk myself as happened before and my wishes were respected.

I found my stay in hospital less pleasant than before, largely I am sure to the different attitude prevailing in the department. Husbands were not given the same involvement and there were no concessions on visiting. The nursery was treated as some kind of Holy of Holies. Access was virtually by invitation only even when your baby was in there. I realise that security is increasingly important but most mothers like to feel that their baby is theirs wherever he or she may be. At the first hospital we were always welcome in the nursery, and could drop baby off in there when going to be away from our bed for any reason. There was always someone there. Here, we had to leave babies by our beds when absent from the wards and there were long periods when the nursery was unattended so I do not see that security was better served.

I found that information on oneself was also harder to obtain. Nobody told me of any potential problem I might have, and subsequently did have, until I was discharged. I then discovered as I watched the midwife fill the discharge sheet that I had 'ragged membranes' and was informed what this meant only when I asked. She seemed surprised that I wanted to know but did tell me that I may pass clots. I feel that this information should have been given to me earlier and without my having to ask. In the event, it led to prolonged bleeding after discharge and a month later, readmission for a D & C. Unfortunately, this also went wrong and I was back in hospital for a week due to a perforated uterus and bowel.

Iain was very upset by his lack of involvement. First time he felt like part of a team event and second time more like a spectator.

Caesarean birth is not something to dread or to feel unfulfilled about. If I have another child, which I do not think I shall, I should certainly have no fears of another Caesarean. I would prefer, however, not to have it at my local hospital which is somewhat awkward. The Consultant informed me that should I have a third, he would then 'tie off my tubes.' I remarked that should he do so, I should probably sue for assault. As my husband and I need AIH to conceive I am at no risk of accidental pregnancy and I do not believe that it is for surgeons to carry out unnecessary procedures. I am told that this is offered, or pushed, to all third time section patients. I believe there is no medical necessity for this point of view.

See picture page 125

CHRISTINE
HOGG

I don't want to be one of 'those' women who go on and on about 'their birth'. I always wanted to be one of 'those' NCT types who take birth in their stride – all raspberry leaf tea and big smocks, but now I know why some people call it the experience of childbirth.

Being a nurse myself I felt prepared . . . but I wasn't. I now wish I hadn't read any books, magazines, etc, but I read them *all*. I was induced at 39 weeks because of high blood pressure, first by breaking my waters and then with a drip – all within an hour of each other. Ross, my gem of a partner, and I would spend hours in those antenatal days debating over the relative merits of Pethidine *v.* gas and air but with a smug self satisfied air of 'well, it's all in the mind anyway,' and hoping we could get by on just the breathing, walking around and baths, I ended up with *everything*! Drugs, drips and a long, protracted labour that even the midwives admitted was horrendous.

We began with breathing as taught in the antenatal classes, went onto the TENS machine and then, all shame and desperation as I wasn't dilating five hours later, I finally conceded and had Pethidine. Ross was hesitant, but when he saw my pain relieved he is now on MY side! I then went for gas and air on top. I remember hallucinating and thinking that some of the nurses who came to check me were angels sent from heaven, and that I was going to die. (My friend had told me that she had been on a 'Coronation Street' trip, i.e., that she had been in the cast!). But it was a lovely pleasant mellow experience close to the feelings of having three quarters of a bottle of red wine on a Friday night after a hard week! But the release!

The doctors and midwives came in from time to time to check me and my hole, and then blamed me for not dilating. The baby was fine, but how can they blame you; don't they realise that you have no control over this? Ross was gradually being chipped away by all this suffering; his love and concern were ground down. I watched him eating cheese and ham sandwiches and drinking Lilt which he hates. The old cliches.

He wanted to be an active supporter but now became a passive observer. It was happening to us, we had no control – the baby would come sometime but it could probably be a week, a year, who cares!

By midnight – I was induced at 11.00am – the doctor (a kind, funny and warm person) decided to bring my baby out by ventouse. He attempted to give me some choice in the matter but life and a cup of tea was all I wanted. With three midwives, a doctor and a ground down husband shouting at me, I had no choice but to push this baby out. I felt like I was in a dark, deep black hole, with everyone else at the top begging me to push. To push that baby out was the most difficult thing I have ever done; it was as if there was nothing else left in the world. I had always vowed never to scream but I screamed with relief and release in between the pushing. At one point I thought that someone had put a traffic cone up my anus. I could not relate to this feeling.

When Joseph was born, Ross said it was a boy and I sat up to see but he was swept away and as Ross said, 'all I saw was a pair of balls flying out of the room.' He was a flat baby as they say, he looked waxy and white to me but also big with huge soft fatty round arms and legs. I remember thinking that I had loved big dimply babies . . . it was half an hour later, 2.00am when the midwife came back to us to say that he was fine, shocked and traumatised and had gone to special care to be observed. I didn't believe them because I'm a nurse and have lied to people myself to shield them from the truth.

Ross and I took a brave, cheerful, blasé approach with each other, protecting one another secretly believing he was really dead or brain damaged, but later by 4.00am we had got to see him, a pretty, quiet chap who looked like my father, sleepy and irritable.

Ross and I then went our separate brave ways, him back home to cry and smoke (he told me three weeks later) and I back to the ward leaving a baby in special care. It was a lonely sleep, needing my husband and baby.

I cried for the next two days, partly because of the pain I was in but also because I had a baby I didn't know or even recognise, that was being looked after by others. My mother came to visit him twice a day and was genuinely overcome with joy over him but I was appalled by her attitude – I could not connect with this baby. I remember the deep anger and torment I felt. I could even go through the motions of looking as if I cared but I didn't. I didn't want to love him because I felt that if he died I would have more to lose, but then I realised that if he died and I hadn't loved him it would be worse. Throughout this private and very solitary pain I felt the blackest guilt that it was actually my fault he was in this state as I had refused to have a Caesarean. Two days later a senior sister took me on the side, slapped me around the face metaphorically speaking and told me he was fine. I cuddled him that night, attached to the monitor and he looked up at me, recognising this strange woman with tears and a runny nose, and all was well. Two days later he was mine to look after out of an incubator and breastfed. By day eight he was home.

The birth experience was similar to the trauma of a bad car crash but it is a private trauma and difficult to share; Ross was emotionally shattered and is wounded to this day, six and a half months later. Fortunately, he has been able to share this experience with other men which has helped. I feel I have come to terms with it but I understand how post-traumatic stress feels, what with flashbacks, nightmares, etc.

Our son, however, is a bright shining light in all this. Despite his traumas he's a placid, happy baby, who loves company and laughs a deep throaty chuckle, throwing his head back in the process. He is normal in every way despite my horror, to the point where sometimes I feel a deep connection that he is older, much older than his six months. He brings us fundamental joy; the attachment and love supersedes everything. I feel as if I have been ravenously hungry for years but that this baby has brought me the feelings of a large calorific meal – it is deeply pleasurable and enormously satisfying.

See picture page 58

It all began on 24th December, Christmas Eve when I went to antenatal clinic for a routine check up. I was 38 weeks and 3 days pregnant and my expected date of delivery was 4th January. I was 19 years old at the time and it was my first baby. The midwife took my blood pressure and told me it was unusually high so she called the doctor in to check me over. I was told I had pre-eclampsia, a killer disease which affects pregnant women and can develop in less than a day. I had all the signs which were raised blood pressure, fluid retention and protein in the urine. Another name for it is pregnancy induced hypertension. I'd had a reasonably healthy pregnancy apart from morning sickness at the beginning and indigestion and backache near the end, so I was shocked to hear I would have to be admitted to hospital straight away. After being admitted and shown where all the facilities were, I was told to have complete bedrest and placed on a foetal monitor after which a doctor came and examined me, checked my baby's heartbeat and position. By this time I was completely devastated at being in hospital on Christmas Eve and when the carol singers came round I wanted to curl up and die.

The following day, Christmas Day, the hospital Consultant came to brief me on what was going to happen. He told me they would have to induce my labour as my blood pressure was getting higher and my condition was worsening. I ended up waiting six days until there was a delivery suite available as the induction had been postponed several times already due to the rush of babies being born over the Christmas period. My condition had deteriorated rapidly over the six days I had waited, which were the longest of my life. So when a midwife came at 5.00am on the morning of 30th December to inform me there was a delivery suite available and I would be taken down in an hour's time to be induced, I was in one way relieved that the waiting was over and I was going to have my baby, but in another I was extremely nervous and frightened of the unknown.

Once in the delivery suite I was given a very unflattering gown to put on. Next to arrive was a midwife who inserted a pessary into the neck of my womb to soften and help dilate the cervix. The midwife then connected me up to a foetal monitor which was something I was used to by now as I had been on it twice a day for the last week. Because I couldn't move around whilst attached to the monitor, I was left lying on the delivery bed while the midwife went to perform various other duties elsewhere. I lay there alone for an hour with only an occasional bleep from the monitor for company and the midwife popping her head around the door from time to time to check the print out readings.

ELAINE GUDGIN

By now I was starting to feel a mild period pain and was experiencing faint contractions. I watched the monitor cautiously reassuring myself I wasn't imagining things. Just as I was beginning to think I had been abandoned, the midwife who had first attended me came back to internally examine me to see if the pessary had worked and whether or not my cervix had started to dilate. It turned out the pessary had not been as successful as hoped so I was taken off the monitor and allowed to go to the toilet which by now was a relief.

Later I discovered the unbelievable comfort of a specially designed beanbag after being carefully lowered onto it by another midwife accompanied by a student midwife. They took turns sitting with me and checked my blood pressure every few minutes chatting casually to help pass the time. I was then asked if I would like some music on to relax me and I decided it would be a good idea, so the midwife proceeded to play my Guns 'n Roses tape. As I looked around the delivery suite the clock caught my eye and I noticed the time was 9.00am. My contractions were beginning to get more frequent and more painful.

My mother had arrived by now to keep me company until my husband finished his shift at work and could be with me. Whilst spending another hour sitting on my marvellous bean bag the midwife did her best to explain what was going to happen next. To start off labour properly they were going to perform a prostin induction, but first my waters would have to be broken by scratching my womb with a specially designed instrument. So by the time a male midwife had arrived I was a little less than enthusiastic and as I was helped back onto the delivery bed I had a good view of the surgical instruments laid out on the trolley he had wheeled in. After the necessary preparation the midwife began. He took what I can only describe as a large crochet hook and inserted it into me until it wouldn't go any further, then he began to break my waters by puncturing the amniotic sac which held my baby. The whole operation was most unpleasant. The pressure was unbearable and the pain was excruciating, so I was relieved when I felt a warm gush of amniotic fluid flood onto the bed.

After being manoevred off the bed I was given another gown to change into. Then I was connected up to the monitor once more and confined to bed. By now I was in absolute agony and was doubled up with the pain. My breathing exercises helped for a while but the contractions were lasting longer and each time the pain was more intense. I asked the midwife if I could have an epidural as I had discussed this with her earlier on. The doctor arrived shortly after with the equipment. I was advised to sit on the edge of the bed and lean over a chair so that my back was arched. The doctor covered my lower back with antiseptic and then began to insert a large needle into my spine. He was having difficulty finding the correct location which is the space between the vertebra called the epidural gap, and had another four attempts all to no avail. By this time the pain was overwhelming and having to keep perfectly still was an impossible task as I was shaking uncontrollably due to high blood pressure which was rapidly rising with the pain.

An onlooking midwife who sympathised with me rushed to my aid with an injection of opiate which is an extremely strong analgesic. I shall be eternally grateful to that woman. Meanwhile, the doctor had sent for a specialist who had been on his day off but was now on his way to the hospital. When he arrived I was still very relaxed and drowsy. Seeing this, the specialist told me to lie on my side and bring my knees up to my chest. This time I couldn't even feel the needle going in and was amazed to learn that the needle had been successfully inserted into my spine in a period of minutes.

I was helped up and made comfortable by two midwives whilst the specialist pumped the anaesthetic into my spine. I was placed back on the foetal monitor while I waited for the epidural to take effect. It was decided that an internal monitor was to be attached to the top of my baby's head to detect any signs of foetal distress, so I was wired up to yet another monitor. Within 10 minutes the epidural had worked and a lovely warm sensation started flowing around my body. I was numb from the waist down, which was its purpose, and soon had no sensation of pain either. The anaesthetic in the epidural was topped up every hour to prevent the pain from returning, so I was able to lie back and rest ready for the next stage.

As I could no longer feel the contractions the midwife had to put her hand on my stomach to feel them and watch the monitor to see how often they were coming. By now my husband had arrived and so my mother left us reluctantly after helping me through the first half. The doctor had brought two drips in now and was busy putting several needles into the back of my hand. The first drip contained a saline solution of sugar and salt in liquid form for energy, and the second contained a synthetic drug called Syntocinon which substitutes the natural drug your body produces to induce labour naturally. The male midwife came every half hour to examine me internally to see how far my cervix had dilated. I wasn't doing as well as he hoped and was only two centimetres dilated. I needed to be 10 centimetres to enable my baby's head to pass through. The drip containing the Syntocinon drug was turned up gradually more and more to speed up my labour as my baby was beginning to show signs of foetal distress and my blood pressure was becoming dangerously high.

I was terribly thirsty by now but was only allowed to suck an ice cube which wasn't exactly thirst quenching. Whilst observing the monitor my husband noticed the readings were starting to go haywire. Alarmed at this he went to alert the midwife who had gone for more ice cubes. After checking the monitor the midwife immediately sent for the doctor. When the doctor arrived he examined the monitor reading and informed me the baby was showing signs of serious foetal distress and had an erratic heart-beat, and if it wasn't born soon it may not survive. The only option was to be transferred to the operating theatre to have an emergency Caesarean section as my own condition was also deteriorating. So the male midwife returned to take a blood sample from my baby's head and gave me another internal examination. The midwife turned to the doctor, then they both approached me and said I was suddenly 10 centimetres dilated and that a Caesarean section wouldn't be necessary, and with a bit of luck the midwife could deliver my baby now. I was so astonished with being told I would have my baby in minutes I just wanted to get it over with.

My baby was lying in what is called the face position which the midwife explained is quite rare as only 0.04 per cent of births are presented in this way. Therefore, the doctor would have to use forceps to help him turn my baby around to the correct position and to assist with the actual birth. I was only allowed to push twice as the doctor feared the strain and the high blood pressure would be too much for my heart. As I'd had an epidural I couldn't move my legs, so to assist the doctor my legs were put in surgical stirrups.

The first push was the hardest and I really had to bear down and push for quite a long time until my baby's head was born. The doctor had to perform an episiotomy to prevent my perineum from tearing in the process. The second push was slightly easier and not as prolonged. After the doctor had delivered my baby he held him up so I could see him for the first time. Then came the final stage of labour which I wasn't so aware of now my baby had been born. The umbilical cord which had been the lifeline to my baby was cut. It had served its purpose. The midwife then proceeded to deliver and examine the placenta which was then hurriedly taken away by a nurse. The midwife's next task was to stitch up my perineum and insert a catheter into my bladder as the doctor had to be certain my kidneys were functioning correctly, and I had previously agreed for a doctor to take samples of my urine to use for research into kidney failure caused by pre-eclampsia. The drip containing the Syntocinon drug was taken out of my hand but the saline drip remained in for two days as I was very weak. The whole event lasted 19 hours 2 minutes from start to finish. My baby was born at 7.02pm on 30th December. When these various tasks were completed my legs were removed from the surgical stirrups and after the midwives had attended my baby I was finally allowed to hold him.

This was the moment I had waited so long for. For nine months I had lived with a bump, something that hiccuped, kicked and wriggled, something that had been a home for my precious baby boy whose beautiful big eyes could melt the coldest heart. I was overwhelmed with emotion. I was so proud of him and when I looked at his father his tears said it all. It was over at last and every moment was worth it to have my adorable baby Elliot.

This was the most traumatic event in my life. I would never have another baby as I couldn't bear to go through it all again and also because I don't honestly think I could love another baby as much as I love my little Elliot.

See picture page 126

TERESA PERRIGO

For my first born I managed to be allowed a home delivery which was very important to me as I wanted to be in control of my own labour and to have minimal interference. My pregnancy was very healthy but throughout I made it clear to the obstetricians that if there was any complication I would not hesitate to come into hospital. However, as long as things were fine I was determined to exercise my right to have the baby how and where I wished, much to the disapproval of the hospital medical fraternity who were aiming for 100 per cent hospitalisation for births in the area and so maximum control over mothers.

This comes from my diary:- Not a wink of sleep for me on Sunday night – really bad low back pains. Tried every position to relieve it without success. Could this be the start of labour? In the morning the pains continued but were also moving round to the front. I telephoned the midwife at 8.00am and asked her advice – she said to see how they progressed. Carl stayed and timed the tightenings – already lasting 45 seconds and occurring every four to five minutes, so we telephoned the midwife again and she said she was on her way.

She arrived at about 11.00 am with another and they brought in all their gear. Then she examined me and said I was already three centimetres dilated. So we all settled down for the labour. Carl was great, making cups of tea and snacks. It took three to four hours for me to dilate another one centimetre and the back pain was still bad. The thought of it taking three to four hours for each further centimetre up to full dilation at 10 centimetres was a bit daunting, so I agreed to have my waters broken. They must have been incredibly tough but eventually they burst and out rushed a torrent of amniotic fluid which took us all by surprise with its quantity. Then the contractions really continued in earnest and were more how I'd imagined they would be, but still with terrible back pains. The midwives were great, massaging my back and helping me into different positions. I took a bath and then another one later on.

By that stage I was seven and a half centimetres dilated, but not coping very well with the back pains. The front pains weren't so bad. I knew I was tensing up and not relaxing with the breathing and I really felt I needed some help so I asked for gas and air. What brilliant stuff!! Apparently, I had a continuous grin on my face after that. It was a great light-headed feeling which just distanced me enough from the intensity of the contractions at front and back. It didn't seem very long before I began to get the urge to bear down. I was checked and found to be fully dilated.

So bear down I did, but all to no avail – the baby appeared to be stuck midway down the birth canal, and the back pains were almost overpowering. I pushed with each contraction. It was very frustrating and it seemed the baby was quite content to stay where it was. By that time it was getting on for 9.00pm (12 hours of labour) and the midwife sensed I was not coping with the back pains very well, so she thought it was better for us to go into hospital in the ambulance.

I was too absorbed by the contractions to be aware of what was happening but apparently instead of sending an ambulance which was really all that was needed since the baby was not in the least distressed, the obstetrician made a political decision to send out the 'flying squad'.

As luck would have it the ambulance which brought them broke down so it took an hour for them to arrive. They all traipsed upstairs – doctor, junior doctor, midwife and ambulance-men. I had a drip put in my hand (yuk!) and was hauled onto a chair stretcher and humped down two flights of stairs and out into the ambulance, still clutching the mouthpiece like a lifeline. The driver must have managed to find every pothole there was on the road to the hospital: however, I was totally involved with breathing and resisting the urge to bear down by breathing away the contractions.

When we reached the hospital I was taken into the delivery room and prepared for a forceps delivery. Local anaesthetic, catheter in bladder (yuk, yuk, yuk!) Thankfully, I couldn't see that much, having my legs up in stirrups and flat on my back. No chance for gravity to play its part now.

Then the dreaded snip of the episiotomy scissors as the routine episiotomy was done. And then the scraping of the forceps blades as they were placed around the head, and then breathe out and push! Wonderful feeling as the head moved down the birth canal. Then I could feel the top of the head as it crowned. Then one more contraction and the head was out. And then a few more and 'it's a little girl!!'

Visions of a little baby, creamy coloured and shiny with vernix, dark-haired and crying. She was put on my belly for a few moments and then whisked off to be cleaned and Apgar tested (8/10 after one minute, 9/10 after five minutes) and weighed – 6lb 13oz. Then she was dressed in a hospital robe, wrapped in the blanket and given to me.

In the meantime the Doctor who was rather heavy handed did the 'sew-up' job. OUCH! Then she was given to me and we were left for 45 minutes in the delivery room. I put her straight to the breast and she began to suckle and Carl took some pictures. The midwife brought us tea and toast.

I was then wheeled to a bathroom and Carl ran me a bath. My legs were like jelly so I needed a deal of assistance from Carl and also I wasn't keen on my baby being left alone for long. We were taken up in the lift to the fourth floor and I was lifted up and lowered onto the bed. Carl had thrown together some things for us which he put in the bedside cupboard. I felt really shivery and cold and asked for a blanket. Carl left to catch a taxi home and I lay there in the darkness unable to sleep in my joy of euphoria. I lifted Blaze out of the plastic fish tank and the two of us slept side by side. Or at least Blaze slept – I was too full of delight and relief to get much sleep. We were greeted by a beautiful sunny morning with a mist gathering over the hills. It really was a 'blaze' of a morning. Breakfast of Weetabix and milk and milky tea was quite frankly the most delicious I could ever remember.

Various tests and checks in the morning. The Consultant came and wagged his finger at me for taking the risks he had warned about in having a home birth first time round. It really was water off a duck's back now that I had Blaze with me.

We had to wait for the anti-D to arrive before I could be discharged, so it was 6 o'clock in the evening before we were able to leave the hospital.

Home! Blaze is so beautiful. I can't believe it's possible to have produced such a perfect little creature. She's so dainty and has beautiful blue eyes and a lovely shaped head. Fortunately, hardly marked at all by the forceps – just a big bruise on the back of her head where she got stuck in my pelvis and a few grazes where she rubbed with the top of her head against my spine and one forceps mark on her left cheek. I was glad to have had most of the labour at home, and given the choice, I would like to have another home birth, though the midwife thought it unlikely I'd be allowed to have my second baby there. The third perhaps!!?

My first pregnancy went extremely well. I worked until a week before, and sat an exam five days before the birth, and felt, apart from the odd niggly pain, healthy and prepared for the birth. I had attended local classes and assumed that there was no reason for the birth to be other than painful but bearable. At my last hospital visit, the Consultant had said everything seemed fine, including the baby's position and we should just wait for the big day.

On the morning of the 30th October I felt some pains and got up early. At 8.30am I went into the kitchen to find a gush of water, warm, running down my legs. I telephoned the hospital and they suggested I should go in. After breakfast and a shower I packed my bag and we went to the hospital thinking this was it! So far, not too bad. On arrival, the normal labour rooms were being decorated so I was taken to a four-bed ward where women in various stages of labour were groaning loudly. I was examined by a midwife and then a none too gentle doctor who muttered that my waters hadn't broken but that I had probably wet myself. I wasn't in the habit of doing this, and was a little surprised when they wanted to admit me if nothing was happening. At this stage I was one and a half centimetres dilated!

I was sent up to a Florence Nightingale ward and Andrew was sent home. The ward was a mixture of women with new babies and those on bed rest. Nothing much happened until about 11.00pm when the pains started in real earnest. Everyone around me was asleep or trying to be and staff were thin on the ground. The pains were all in my back. The classes I had been to didn't prepare me for this. All the time I was conscious of trying not to wake other people and wishing Andrew was there with me. The only position I was vaguely comfortable in was all fours on the bed. Other mums came to see if I was OK so I must have been groaning. A Sister examined me and I was no more dilated, so she couldn't yet send me to the delivery room. The pain was very wearing and I felt very alone and constrained by circumstances, wishing I was at home. Occasionally, an auxiliary rubbed my back. I was told that the baby was in a posterior position and that it causes backache labour. I wasn't told that walking around would help things, nor did anyone suggest any form of relief – I lie, I was offered two paracetamol.

Eventually, after some hours, I could stand it no longer. I needed to move and decided to walk to the toilets. There I promptly vomited and my legs were shaking, making me feel unsteady. The Sister re-examined me and found I was seven centimetres. At last I could go to the delivery room. This was

DAWN
ROBINSON-WALSH

about six thirty in the morning and I was glad that it would all soon be over. I was not offered gas and air but was given Pethidine. I fell asleep. Andrew was there when I woke. The Pethidine left me feeling out of control and drowsy.

Eventually, after much monitoring, I was taken to the delivery room. The elderly midwife wasn't very friendly, the doctor was hard to understand because he mumbled and was extremely brusque. A student doctor stayed, with my permission, and he was great, telling me I was doing well and holding my hand. Andrew was told to stay at the head of the bed and had to help to contort me into all sorts of positions in an attempt to turn the baby. I seemed to be pushing ineffectively for ages and was exhausted. By now I was wired up to a drip, had a catheter inserted and an internal monitor on the baby's head.

The doctor decided on forceps due to foetal distress and prolonged second stage. No one told me what was happening although my main concern was to get the baby out; I'd had enough. I later read in my notes I suffered maternal distress. This irked me because I thought I'd been extremely calm but discovered it meant exhaustion rather than a delicate mental state. My husband noticed the changes in the baby's heartbeat on the monitor which had him worried; luckily, I missed it. He also had the misfortune to notice the doctor struggling to assemble the forceps which didn't inspire confidence.

As far as I was concerned, a kind word or explanation would have been nice, but perhaps everyone was too busy with the action. An episiotomy was administered. The forceps were used and they shouted at me to push. Eventually, (minutes) out rushed a baby at quite some speed; I'd begun to think it would never come out. I saw a mass of cord and in my dazed state announced, slightly disappointedly, 'Oh, it's a boy.' 'No, it's a girl,' they replied without any sense of joy. She was whisked away and examined by a paediatrician on standby but had an Apgar score of nine at five minutes and was fine. I was left. Andrew asked if he could nip out for some air – I think he'd found it rather gruelling. She was born at 11.58am 31st October. The doctor then decided to suture me. It hurt a great deal, just when I'd thought it was all over. He told me I was being unco-operative because I was tensing but I couldn't help it. I found his manner totally unacceptable but was too weak to make a stand. He called the Consultant who decided to suture me under general anaesthetic pointing out it was 'on humanitarian grounds' for which I was eternally grateful. I honestly believe if the doctor had continued to suture me, I would never have had more children.

I woke up feeling lousy with a drip in place and an extremely sore perineum. I felt geriatric compared to the 19 year old in the next bed when I fould I could hardly walk. My episiotomy had extended and I had sustained quite bad tearing requiring some continuous internal suturing and a few external stitches. Luckily, the Consultant made a good job of the suturing (I dread to think what his assistant would have done) and after 12 weeks I was more or less as good as new.

Despite the discomfort following, I took to my daughter, Alexandra Jennie, immediately, all 6lb 6oz of her. She wasn't objectively speaking beautiful with her mousy hair and forceps marks, but I was enthralled by her. She breastfed beautifully, once the Pethidine had worn off – she was very drowsy for two days. The delivery had not been easy, and I felt a little guilty about my seeming incompetence (feelings I later exorcised), but I still feel resentful that the staff involved did not handle it sensitively on the whole. Everything seemed to go wrong from stepping through the hospital door – had the junior doctor and midwife concerned had a modicum of training in bedside manner, I feel a difficult situation would have been made easier. Obviously, though, I remain grateful to them for delivering me a healthy baby.

My son, Laurence Stephen, was born 19 months later. They were close together because I felt if I left it too long I'd never do it again! I booked into a different hospital because of my psychological feelings about the first. My GP did tell me that he had known women who had had horrendous first time deliveries have a subsequent baby with no problem, but I have to say I didn't believe him. When I was taken in to be induced, I was fearful, and was dreading the birth anyway. However, I felt more prepared (having attended NCT classes this time). Labour went like a textbook description. (I had prostaglandin gel inserted but was already three centimetres). The young midwife was friendly and empathetic. I could labour in private with my husband and used TENS and in stage two some gas and air. The pushing went on for a while (this does not seem to be my strong point), and Laurence was delivered onto my stomach when I eventually felt the mystical urge to push that I hadn't encountered before. The best news was, apart from a healthy baby, that I only had a slight scratch and needed no stitches. The difference afterwards was tremendous. I felt very high, Andrew and I both enjoyed the birth much more, and the staff were really helpful and positive. A totally different experience.

See pictures page 60

GILLIAN BECK

I am 30 years old and Helen is my first baby. I have had multiple sclerosis for 12 years. This causes weakness, mainly in my right leg, poor balance and lack of stamina. I walk with crutches for limited distances and use a wheelchair when tired. Both my GP and my specialist expressed no worry about me becoming pregnant, as it was unlikely to affect the course of the disease, which was my main worry at the start.

The Consultant I saw at the antenatal clinic didn't think I'd have any problems giving birth but was concerned that I might become overtired if I had a long labour. Because of this, he suggested I had an epidural, but said it was entirely up to me whether I decided to have it or not. He also recommended ventouse extraction in case I didn't have the strength to push the baby out.

I wanted a birth with as little intervention as possible, partly because I was worried about the effect any drugs would have on my MS and partly because I know my own limitations – with an epidural I wouldn't be in control. I find it very easy to relax, so I wasn't too concerned about becoming overtired or about coping with labour pains.

Because Helen was overdue I was going to be taken in to be induced but luckily my contractions started the day before I was due to go in. I'd been to antenatal classes and read all the books and I planned to go into hospital when my contractions were 10 minutes apart. However, after the first hour they were coming every three minutes. At around midnight I went into second stage labour and the contractions faded away to such an extent that I had to be put on a drip to encourage me to push.

I went to hospital as I didn't know what to make of the length of time between contractions. I felt rather foolish when I was found to be only one centimetre dilated. I was sent up to a ward as the midwife thought nothing much would happen that night. However, by the end of visiting time I was five and a half centimetres so was sent back down to the delivery suite.

I didn't need any pain relief and managed to stay quite relaxed just sitting in a chair. I felt no inclination to move about like I had planned. By 11.30pm my neck was aching with sitting so long and when I got onto the bed the midwife examined me and was amazed to find I was fully dilated and she could see the baby's head. Even though my contractions virtually stopped, Helen's head moved down the birth canal with very little help from me.

With only a couple of centimetres left to go, and no sign of her moving, the doctor used ventouse extraction and Helen came out in just a few seconds. I only needed two stitches as Helen had her hand on her head and caused a small tear. I felt elated. I wasn't at all tired and I'd had the kind of labour and birth that I'd wanted. The next day I felt so well I wanted to go home there and then.

Although I had no medication during labour I have very little recollection of things that happened. I'm glad my husband was there as he can remind me and tell me about things I just didn't notice. I think labour is so overwhelming, even if it is fairly pain-free as mine was, and that all the little things you think will be important beforehand just pale into insignificance.

SERGA COLLETT

My husband and I had been thinking of an addition to our family for some years but more recently had taken it seriously; so after a year of trying I went to see a specialist. After a number of tests he suggested a laparoscopy, the result of which however was something I hadn't expected. As I came out of the general anaesthetic he asked: 'Did your mother take any drugs while she was pregnant with you?' Well, how was I to know? So diligently I went back to my mother and asked 'Mom . . .' and indeed the answer was 'yes', while she was pregnant with me she had an attack of TB and was advised to abort me, but against the doctor's orders decided to continue the pregnancy (thank goodness!) so she was given drugs to keep the illness in check. The result anyway is that I have something called a bicornute uterus, basically it means that my uterus has two sides like the shape of a heart rather than the normal pear shape. This does not prevent getting pregnant but it does make it more difficult and the pregnancy too is a bit more traumatic. Anyway, following this great discovery, the month following the laparoscopy 'bingo' that little blue strip of paper turned pink and our excitement knew no bounds. What a pregnancy too – I wasn't sick, no heartburn, no piles or indeed anything that my friends complained of. I did start bleeding at eight weeks – panic – but an ultrasound showed no problems. (I was later told that this is quite common at four, eight and 12 weeks).

I was seen frequently by my specialist who also fortunately is a Consultant of the hospital. I felt a little bit like a VIP – whenever I came in, I was shown to all the medical students who had to diagnose my condition. From week 24, I was advised that the baby could arrive at any time – I suppose due to the lack of space in the uterus – and every time I inched away from home very gingerly, I didn't fancy trying to explain my medical history to some strange doctor in some strange hospital. I felt and still feel in the best hands locally. Ruth held on in there – we had plenty of ultrasound scans and because she stayed breech in just the one half of my heart-shaped uterus (I think the lack of space made it impossible for her to turn), so she was definitely going to have to arrive by Caesarean.

During my 36 week check, the Consultant said: 'Well, what are you doing on the 19th February?' and that is how my baby's birthday was decided.

On February 18th, I dutifully arrived at the hospital and felt like a spare part – I even helped the midwives rearrange the flowers. Things got going however in the evening, I was monitored – very worrying – whenever the monitor slips or the baby moves the heartbeat of course no longer registers on the machine – and then came the worst part of the whole Caesarean – I was shaved down below! I just hadn't thought about it – and I just gawped at the midwife when she came in with a razor! Eventually the 19th dawned, my husband arrived and I was wheeled up to the operating theatre for 9.00am – then they prepared me for the epidural. The anaesthetist and his assistant were smashing and we had a really good laugh while the epidural started to take effect, so much so that the next Caesarean case waiting outside heard me giggle and told me afterwards decided that it couldn't be as bad as all that after all. In fact I have photos of me holding the epidural needle with a big smile on my face and one of my husband all gowned up and giggling. I must admit, as I was wheeled into the operating theatre, I did have great misgivings about my choice of having an epidural but when I didn't feel the first incision I relaxed. Ten minutes passed whilst the anaesthetist gave me a running commentary on what was happening (you cannot see anything that is happening) – a slurping sound as the amniotic fluid drained off, then a 'please push' and my little girl arrived at 10.23am, weighing a good 7lb 6oz at 38 weeks.

It took a lot longer to sew me up than it took to open me up, but I was mesmerized by my husband holding little Ruth with the February sun shining on their faces. How very lucky I was! (I couldn't hold Ruth myself as my hands were squashed underneath my chin whilst they were working down below.) As I was wheeled into the recovery room I was given Ruthie to hold for the first time. What perfection – I was overawed. I stayed in hospital for five days – I walked for the first time the next day but by the end of the week I was fit, and by the time I went home, I was no more sore than any other Mom who had just given birth.

I hear so many horror stories about Caesareans and indeed had been frightened by them myself, that I want to let anyone who has the prospect of having one know – it is a very special experience – to witness with your partner the most important event of your life and with no pain (that comes later but is bearable). As for the scar – that is no longer visible because of the positioning of the cut on the bikini line.

See picture page 129

YVONNE WHEELER

At 36½ years old and with my first pregnancy, the obstetrician wanted to whisk me in for induction within three days of due date 'because he always did with his older first-timers', which seemed a poor reason given that everything else was fine. I felt well, no blood pressure problems and no oedema; the pregnancy had been quite normal, although very trying for the first five months with constant queasiness but no sickness: the further it progressed, the better I felt. So we opted to wait for Nature – with the community midwife keeping an eye on me. An examination nine days overdue found the cervix was ripening, so we tried internal stretching, bumpy car rides, etc. to encourage it along, to no effect, so three days later, Sunday, we reported to the Maternity Ward for induction at 3.00pm. Went through admission checks, was monitored and examined – one centimetre dilated with soft cervix – and was allowed out for the evening, ostensibly for a last dinner à deux. Back in at 10.00pm and given prostaglandin pessary at 11.00pm. Husband went home, I went to sleep.

Monday

3.30am – woke with backache and a show.

6.30am – cervix stretched and second pessary given

By 9.30am contractions were frequent but irregular – and painfully in my back, which came as a surprise. Padded up and down corridors, leaning over trolley or radiator during contractions, rotating hips, etc. After a bath around noon, contractions were coming every two to five minutes, the pain still mostly in the back.

1.30 pm – examined and assessed at three centimetres dilation, moved into labour ward contractions now every two to three minutes but breathing through them successfully.

2.00pm – restricted to bed for monitoring for '15 minutes', which stretched to an hour and then again at 3.30pm. Contractions more painful while on my back, though watching monitor helped to time breathing to best effect; much easier moving around, sitting on edge of bed or on pouffe or leaning over table. Even fell asleep for about 20 minutes!

6.00pm and the beginning of the end when I had to lie on my back for another internal examination – only four centimetres – a one centimetre gain in four hours, which wasn't fast enough. After discussion with midwife and doctor, agreed to ARM and, more reluctantly, to the immobility of a dextrose drip to counteract the dehydration identified from ketones found in urine.

6.15pm – ARM done and meconium found in the waters, a sign of potential foetal distress, so hooked back on to monitor – reassuring strong and steady heart beat. But now the back pain from being on the bed was more than the breathing could override.

Tried Entonox – sick! all over the bed. By the time this was sorted out, being rolled back and forth for new sheets between contractions, which were even stronger now after the ARM, I was exhausted and in agony. An epidural was the only answer to kill the pain – drugs to take the edge off would not have been enough – so the anaesthetist was sent for. A long painful hour of waiting for his arrival and discussing the procedure left me too weak to sign the consent form, so hubby obliged. Finally wheeled into a small theatre, after being crashed into the wall *en route*, in a very sorry state, moaning and/or screaming quietly as the contractions came. Curling into a ball was neither easy nor compatible with the contractions and the first attempt failed to allow the tube to be fed in properly. Advice was offered from an ungowned stranger standing at the door (who later proved to be the senior anaesthetist) and so:

8.00pm – peace at last, pain steadily reducing until no feeling. Dead legs but toes could wiggle. Wheeled back, without crashing, to 'our' room and hooked back on to monitor to find contractions now lasting two minutes out of every four.

10.00pm – new examination, now seven to eight centimetres. Great elation that at least some progress was being made, though still on slow side. Feeling was returning though, and much faster than expected, so in pain again while anaesthetist was tracked down for a top-up (found in Casualty theatre!) before the welcome sensation of cold trickling down my back and, ten minutes later, no more pain again, just a bit of tingling in face.

11.00pm – visited by paediatrician to explain she'd have to clean out baby's lungs before allowing normal respiration to be sure that no meconium had got into them – so no delivery on to tummy: another hope dashed.

Tuesday

12.15 am – epidural again wearing off, so another examination – only the same dilation as before. Great disappointment as we'd expected this to be it – had been on monitor for four hours with strong and regular contractions, no foetal distress. Talked into Oxytocin by the doctor who explained that we must make progress before I had no strength left.

1.00am – second top up of epidural

1.30am – more dextrose and Oxytocin set up – another machine for hubby to watch. At least it helped keep him awake between the cups of coffee. Dose steadily increased over the next three hours, with a third epidural top up around 3.00am.

4.30am – big examination as the epidural wore off with midwife calling Sister for help. Only six centimetres and now very swollen and inflamed. Ticked off for not knowing what the 'Sagittal suture' was (we'd known of everything else!)

5.00am – big discussion outside (and inside between us) on whether time had come for a Caesarean. I'd been going for 24 hours and we were both exhausted.

At last doctor came in and tentatively suggested the Caesarean – agreed instantly as long as it could be done under epidural and with husband present and in the meantime PLEASE, PLEASE TOP UP THE EPIDURAL. He did.

Theatre readied, hubby changed into green suit, very nervous and emotionally drained but hanging in there for me.

6.00am (ish) – into theatre and to nice chatty anaesthetist, slapping on sticky labels to heart and shoulders to monitor heart rate, blood pressure set up on arm and inflatable 'boots' on both legs to maintain circulation. Finally added yet further epidural anaesthetic, tilting operating table from side to side (with me strapped on yet hanging on in fear of sliding off!) to ensure a good spread of anaesthetic.

No sensation at all of operation – it had started before I had realised – although sound of snipping scissors rather disconcerting. Screen right across chest, so totally 'blind' although husband, sitting at side of my head could watch (or not!).

Head emerged – amazing experience, said hubby, seeing the dirty brown slimy head (from meconium) pulled from the five inch cut – paediatrician at work sucking almost before the rest of the babe appeared.

6.30am – given as time of birth – baby out, with a couple of whimpers and whisked off to be cleaned and tested. Two Apgar tests done – scored six then nine. IT'S A BOY and all OK. Given to Dad to show Mum. Then weighed in at 10lb 4oz – we thought they were kidding. Babies don't come that big. This one did!! Poor little head moulded from pressure against cervix that couldn't let it through.

All stitched up over next 30 minutes or so to chorus of swab counts and wheeled back to our room again. Baby given blood test for sugar levels because of his size, then stomach washed out, while I was being drip fed blood and glucose – though would have preferred a cup of tea.

8.30am – breakfast for Dad and huge sigh of relief that it was all over.

Jamie Martin – welcome to the world! 19th February.

See picture page 127

Towards the end of my pregnancy we became increasingly certain that I wouldn't go to full term (March 10th) as I felt that there wasn't much room left inside, and I'd started snapping at Paul (he declared my hormones were getting back to normal!). I felt very fit and active, out every day and swimming 40 lengths twice a week if I could find the time. So, on March 1st I set off to town to go shopping.

It was annoying to have to walk a long distance to the shops from my car, unusual for me to worry about this, but I became aware of increasing pressure on my pelvis as the morning wore on, perhaps the head was engaging? I'd lost weight at the last clinic, so suspected something might be happening. Driving back down the motorway I became aware of tightenings and pressure in the bump area – Braxton Hicks? There hadn't been any before – so I began to time them – very gentle, every 10 minutes. Told Paul at lunchtime, we both felt no need to do anything about it. So, I went swimming that afternoon, my normal 40 lengths, wondering whether anything would actually happen as these continued. I felt fine.

By late afternoon they were still happening, no pain, but the bump visibly tightened about every 10 minutes. Finally, at 8.15pm my waters went with a gush and the plug appeared. Now we knew we were in business. The contractions grew stronger, were irregular, but at less than 10 minute intervals. We rang my community midwife (who had offered to deliver me) and she told us to ring back when we wanted her to come and examine me. I was then attached to the TENS machine we had rented and it provided a lot of help throughout the early hours of labour. We watched TV and I had a long soak in the bath (even though my waters had gone, the midwife said that my bath would be clean enough). By 10.30pm things had strengthened, but were no closer together or regular, so Midwife came to examine me. The internal was painful, surprisingly, and all others that night were unpleasant, particularly in the later stages. She couldn't reach my cervix, but confirmed that we were in business. She went home to bed, having arranged that the hospital should ring her as soon as we were admitted.

By now I was squatting through contractions, even in the bath, and by 1.00am I felt ready to go to hospital as the contractions were now much stronger, and I spent the 30 minute journey on all fours on the back seat of the car. Ironically, as it turned out, we took the baby seat with us in hopeful anticipation of doing a 'domino' and coming home that evening!! I remember looking at it and finding it hard to believe that we would actually have a baby

JOSIE MARTIN

to put into it soon.

I had to squat through a contraction at the door of the delivery building, much to the amusement of passing staff. The midwife arrived soon after. Throughout the night I really lost all sense of time – Paul tells me that it seemed much longer to him than it did to me! The midwife is a wonderful lady, and it was wonderful to have a known, sensible face that we could utterly rely on. She and Paul rubbed my back all night, she brought in mattresses, sheets, bean bags, birthing stools – you name it! I didn't want to go near a bed, didn't like leaning up against things upright, and was much happier squatting, or kneeling across Paul's knees as he sat in a chair, my head in his stomach, so I was cuddled and rubbed at the same time. That contact was terribly important and their enthusiastic support and reminders to breathe through the worst was really helpful and positive.

I was quickly onto gas and air which helped, but made me feel a bit sick at first. We soon sussed out how to use it in anticipation of the contractions. The midwife found that I had a 'lip' on my cervix and for what seemed like ages I had to puff-puff-blow at the height of contractions to stop the desire to push which began around 4.30am. As Paul puts it 'the awful noises started'! It was very comforting to bellow and grunt, and it didn't seem to be me making the noises. It was painful as the midwife kept having to push the lip back during contractions – that was a really hard time as they came very close together. Amazingly, I didn't swear once!!

After that, and lying on my side on the beanbag, at last I was allowed to push. At first we seemed to get somewhere, but it seemed I wasn't pushing effectively, and to make matters worse, the contractions began to weaken and diminish in number. We tried the birthing stool, but by 7.00am the midwife was suggesting the birthday bed in stirrups. I was past caring and simply wanted the baby out. A doctor was called in and a drip set up – after which the contractions returned with increasing strength, intensity and pain – and still no baby! At 8.15am my midwife had to disappear to do a clinic, Paul was wrecked and upset, I was in a good deal of pain and she clearly hated going. Luckily her replacement was super.

By now I was shaking with trauma and pain, and the room filled up as the decision was made to give me an epidural (yes, please!). For 30 minutes I virtually blacked out as I had to stay still while it took effect – that was by far the worst part as the contractions were very strong, I had lost direction and didn't know what to do with them. Awful! Then, bliss, the epidural took effect, and Paul describes being able to finally prize the gas tube out of my hand. The sun was shining and I began to realise that there were at least eight people in the room. We were to be really impressed by the way the staff dealt with us, they explained that they couldn't fit in the forceps, so would try a Ventouse delivery with me pushing. No luck, OK, only option now was a Caesarean. We were quite happy for that to happen, but I wanted to stay awake with the epidural. This was very carefully topped up while I was shaved (I didn't care . . .). Paul appeared, gowned up and we went into theatre. I asked not to be told what was happening (would faint) but chatted aimlessly and watched the sunshine through the roof lights and clung to Paul's hand. It was really happy – it makes me smile to remember it now. I heard a baby but had felt nothing, then Sophie was handed to Paul, all wrapped up, and he held her beside my head.

Wonderful, all those blonde curls, and wide open eyes, it was hard to believe it had finally happened. Paul says that it took at least 30 minutes to stitch me up, I don't remember. He watched it all without letting me know, and was quite traumatized later that day when he thought about what he'd seen. The time in the recovery room afterwards was lovely, quiet and calm, just us and the midwife who washed Sophie, then gave me a wash with my own wash things and chatted. We remembered to take photos, it was a calm and happy relief in the sunshine after a long night.

Looking back, we both feel that the labour was handled exactly as we had wanted, even at the end when they had to step in. Apparently my pelvis was too narrow to allow Sophie through – a somewhat unexpected development with my size eight feet and six foot frame! I have no sense of failure and no fears about another Caesarean, it was such a positive experience. I was pretty shattered over the next weeks, but it was well worth it.

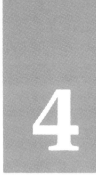

4

HOME AND WATER BIRTHS

Most births take place in hospital but we wanted to devote some space to home birth and water birth which is still relatively unusual. One of the home deliveries was unexpected and quick but most were planned and carried out in conjunction with community midwives. For balance, the assisted delivery section contains an account of a home birth which wasn't straightforward but most contained in this chapter worked well for the mothers concerned. All the women here felt happy about delivering at home but were prepared to go to hospital if necessary.

'**Y**ou fancy a home birth then, do you Susan?' asked my midwife, as she sat sipping coffee amidst the packing cases on her first visit to our new home. We had moved in the previous day, four days before Christmas and two weeks before our second baby was due. Gary had started a new job in Manchester in September: I had opted to stay behind with Luke (then one and a half) and my rapidly expanding five month bump until we'd found a new house.

Suddenly, faced with the fact that I really could choose to have a home delivery with the complete support of midwife and doctor, I felt indecision and uncertainty. The alternative was a short stay in the local hospital with my midwife delivering the baby. She left me to discuss it with Gary but really it didn't take us long to decide that a home birth was what we both wanted.

There were several reasons why we felt that a home delivery was best for us. Luke's delivery, in hospital, though normal had been lengthy and Gary and I both found the hospital environment, the smell, the machines, the long white corridors, strange and alien. Though I have nothing but praise for the midwife who delivered Luke, I am certain that being in a strange place when I was in pain only heightened my anxiety as labour became established, lessening my belief in myself and my feelings of being in control. We wanted something different this time, something more personal and intimate. After all the upheaval and strain of the previous months, re-establishing ourselves as a family and settling Luke in our new home were immensely important to us. We did not want the disruption of spending time, albeit a few hours, in a hospital we'd never visited before. Nor did we want to introduce our son, who we felt had been through much uncertainty and change, to the baby in yet another new strange place.

So . . . the decision was made. I had misgivings, of course I did, but through all the 'what ifs' and 'I'll never forgive myselfs' my midwife was really positive. We had confidence in her from the start. Then came the planning. Through hearsay I'd formed the belief that a home birth was a 'messy' business; that that which is clinically disposed of or cleaned in the hospital laundry can make a disaster area of one's bedroom carpet and bed linen. (Gary didn't feel he could cope with disposing with the afterbirth but the midwife reassured him she'd deal with it).

I visited my Doctor who scanned the baby as a final check that everything was OK. I readily agreed that if my midwife became at all concerned at any time during my labour, then she would call an ambulance before consulting me! This seemed only common sense.

SUSAN SALMON

My midwife inspected and approved the proposed site. There needed to be adequate access to the bed. Then we set about acquiring one plastic sheet to protect the mattress (she suggested I put this on in advance but sleeping was difficult enough by this time without re-creating sauna conditions), two buckets, some oldish bed sheets to deliver onto and lots and lots of newspaper to spread on the floor. The local press became more than just our insight into the goings on in our new home community or as fodder for the local recycling skip.

With everything ready – well, as ready as things could be with full packing cases still packed in the garage – there was nothing to do but wait and hope that when things did get underway we'd be able to get hold of our midwife. Even if for some reason she couldn't come, I would still be able to have a home delivery as there would be a midwife on call. But the relationship I'd built up with her in just a very few weeks was so good that I found it hard to imagine our baby being delivered by anyone else – we REALLY hoped she would be there.

I had a false alarm on 8th January – my midwife visited twice but the contractions never became established. My EDD, 9th January, passed. Just after midnight on 14th I woke with a strong contraction. I dozed until about 2.30am and then when sleep became impossible I woke Gary and rang the midwife. I walked about downstairs, the contractions getting stronger, then fading. She arrived and examined me at about 3.30am. My cervix was three centimetres dilated, thinned out and anterior – this at last was it! Only three centimetres – I remember feeling extremely disappointed and disheartened by that small sounding amount. It had taken me a further 12 hours to fully dilate from that point with Luke, but I consoled myself – at least I was at home and could fill the time as I wished.

The contractions continued to increase in intensity and get closer together. I found the most comfortable position was to kneel on the floor with my head and arms resting on a stool. She monitored the contractions by feeling my abdomen, she took my blood pressure and listened to the baby's heartbeat with a wooden penar (so much warmer than metal ones). This was the only monitoring I experienced during my labour. Luke, by this time wide awake and determined to be part of this early morning action, emptied his night-time drink all over his bed in a final bid to gain the attention of his preoccupied parents. About 3.45am Gary rang friends who were to look after Luke. While waiting for her to arrive, Luke toddled downstairs to play with his toys. My memories of those early hours are dominated by the 'ping pang' of his garage lift – a great distraction from the increasingly intense contractions. I remember my midwife putting her hand on my back and saying, 'you seem really calm and in control Susan; I bet you don't feel that way inside.' She was right and I felt so grateful for her insight and understanding. So far the breathing techniques were just about doing the trick. Luke left at about 5.00am. As I lay on the settee, face pressed into the cushions trying to concentrate absolutely on other things, my friend put her hand on my shoulder and said they'd be thinking of me.

After they'd gone my midwife examined me. I was seven centimetres. I felt that I wanted to lie on the bed but wondered how on earth I could achieve the seemingly impossible feat of climbing the stairs. I made a dash for it between contractions and when I was comfortable on the bed with Gary beside me I asked for some gas and air; she set this up and I started using it at 5.45am. It helped immediately and the knack of timing its use for maximum effect came back. It helped me through the next very difficult half hour when I felt and said to Gary that I couldn't cope with the intensity of the contractions much longer. My midwife tried to break my membranes but they were too well applied to the baby's head; with Luke I'd never experienced the famed primitive, uncontrollable urge to push and I must confess I didn't really experience it this time either, rather a change in emphasis in pressure (as if I needed to go to the loo). I said I thought I wanted to push and after a quick look she found I was fully dilated – this was 6.20am. I found sitting, hugging my knees the most effective and comfortable position in which to push. My waters ruptured spontaneously at 6.30am. It felt great when I felt that head stop sliding back at the end of each contraction and then to put my hand down and touch that very hairy little head, knowing then that this bit (it was then I remembered why it's called labour) was thankfully nearly over.

Unlike Luke whose body slithered out rapidly immediately after his head was delivered, this baby's shoulders got a little stuck. Gary said he could see that little mouth opening in an attempt to wail, but with arms clamped firmly down it was impossible to draw breath. That only lasted a few moments and then at 6.37am our baby made a complete entry into the world and was lifted on to my tummy for us to discover together that we had a beautiful and very noisy daughter.

Bryony Jayne weighed 9lb 5oz and within moments of delivery she breastfed really contentedly. It was really wonderful to be all three of us together in our own bedroom with no need for Gary to rush off and with all the time in the world to touch and hold her.

The third stage of labour lasted 15 minutes but I was far too preoccupied to pay much attention. Thankfully, I had not torn and was spared the discomfort of stitches. The midwife washed the remaining vernix from Bryony's black hair, dressed her and snuggled her into her carrycot, then ran a bath for me. That bath was beyond description: I felt really well, on a tremendous high, better I'm sure than I did two weeks after Luke's birth. While I soaked, viewing my deflated wrinkly tummy, Gary and the midwife changed and re-made the bed and then made toast and tea for us all. She stayed for about an hour or so, writing up notes and checking Bryony and I. After she left, Gary got back into bed, we lifted Bryony in too and the three of us snuggled up and went to sleep. It was wonderful.

After lunch Gary went to fetch Luke. He was rather surprised by the small being wrapped in a shawl and by Mummy's baggy 'flat' tummy but delighted by the racing car tucked inside Bryony's cot for him.

It felt as though Bryony was integrated into our home and family, our daily lives in a gentler and more natural manner because there had been no need to disrupt the continuity of my pregnancy and antenatal care as there had been at the time of Luke's birth. Gary and I both preferred this experience by far and will hopefully be able to enjoy another home delivery in the future. I hope – we both hope – that our experience will perhaps encourage someone else to choose to have their baby at home and that it will be as positive and joyful an experience as Bryony's birth was for us.

I have two boys, Alexander and Nicholas. In most respects they were 'normal' births; they were unusual in that I booked a home birth each time.

JUDY MERRY

I first became pregnant at the age of 36. I suppose I was pretty scared of the idea of labour. I'd had long enough to hear 100 horror stories and I don't think the reality could have been worse than my fears.

From being a small child I have been afraid of hospitals but it didn't occur to me that there was any alternative to a hospital birth. At least not until the consultant told me where I would be having my baby. Being so 'elderly' it would have to be the large consultant unit 10 miles away. I had had every intention of going there but I found myself saying I would like to discuss this and maybe even have a choice? He said he could stop me going to the local hospital. Then I heard myself saying, 'Maybe, but you can't stop me having it at home.'

There were many reasons which made me eventually decide that, for me, this was the right choice. I read every book on pregnancy I could get my hands on before going to my GP and telling him what I'd decided. There is no other doctor I know who at my age would have agreed to this. He was backing his conviction that problems can happen anywhere and that birth at home was no more dangerous than hospital.

I went into labour with Alex five days before the due date. I remember being amazed at how calm I felt. By rights I should have been scared witless, not only by the unknown experience but also the fear of something going wrong and people blaming the home birth.

In fact, something did go wrong. The baby's heart rate dropped and after some debate I was taken to the hospital. There had always been an understanding between myself and the GP that in such circumstances there would be no argument: I would trust his judgement. I can remember sitting alone in the ambulance – my husband was asked to follow in his car – convinced that the baby had already died.

Undoubtedly the worst thing about my first labour was the fear. The contractions weren't easy to cope with. I remember thinking how do people manage if they have learnt no techniques, no confidence in their ability to stay in control. But it was the fear engendered, not by all, but by some of the staff, which I found the worst. A doctor would come into the room, look at the monitor screen, tut-tut to himself and walk out. I said to a sympathetic midwife, 'What is it? Is the baby alright?' She said, 'Yes, fine'.

Altogether labour lasted about 12 hours. That is something which would have horrified me beforehand but I felt it was quite well paced. You forget that contractions are not continuous. The final stages weren't easy with what seemed like a dozen people all throwing in their suggestions, but the baby was loud and healthy. The mother felt a bit battered and would have cheerfully murdered for a cup of tea.

My amenable GP was somewhat startled when 18 months later at the age of almost 39, I became pregnant again and said I wanted this one at home too. His words were, 'Didn't the last experience put you off?' My neighbour – pregnant and a midwife – said she thought I was crazy. But neither my first experience, nor what I had read about home v. hospital made me change my mind. There are many myths about home birth. One is that you will feel really relaxed as you are on your own territory. Well, you do feel more in control, but no-one tells you about the urge to be hospitable. There you are between contractions trying to offer the midwives tea and biscuits.

I went into labour about 9.00pm and we called the midwives about 11.00pm. Those midwives who do home births tend to be older and very confident in their knowledge. I knew that if they had any doubts I would have been taken to the main hospital, but I also knew that they believed in normal birth and that it would not be a decision taken lightly. We all sat round drinking tea and eating lemon cake for an hour or so, me included between contractions. When these got fiercer we went upstairs. Like good midwives they did a lot of watching and monitoring but very little interfering.

I have often thought that there are similarities between labour and seasickness. There is a terrible lethargy. You know you should be shifting position but you just cannot be bothered. I heard them muttering about an episiotomy. I moved! The other low spot was when suddenly the contractions stopped. I had had no pain relief and I thought I couldn't bear another contraction. Then, of course, I was worried that the baby would never come out. The older midwife stood at the end of the bed, hands on her hips and said, 'Well, I've seen thousands of babies come into the world and this one will come out when its ready.' Within a minute the contractions started and 10 minutes later Nicholas was born. I had no stitches, just a bit of bruising. The midwives gave me a bed bath, had a cup of tea and slipped away. It was 4.30am.

My husband crashed out. Alexander was asleep in the other room. I fed Nicky and he crashed out. So I was sitting up in bed, wide awake and feeling high, with no one to help me celebrate.

My baby was a much wanted child. We had been trying for a baby for 10 years, I finally became pregnant and loved every moment of my pregnancy and labour. My baby was due on 6th September. I woke at 9.20am on Sunday, 14th August with pains. I couldn't sit or lie as it was too uncomfortable, so I just kept walking around the house. I left my partner in bed as it was his first day off in five months. My 14 year old niece was staying with me. I thought I'd have a long labour and it was too early for me to go into hospital.

After four hours of walking around the house everything started happening. My waters ruptured and I had and incredible urge to bear down. I was walking along the landing to tell my niece to tell Charlie (my partner) to phone for an ambulance when I had my show. I put my hand underneath me and could feel my baby's head. So I shouted for Charlie to ring for an ambulance and for the district midwife as the baby was arriving. I got myself to the toilet and sat on the very edge so I wouldn't hurt my baby. I put my legs one on each side of the doorway. I delivered my baby's head, then one shoulder, then the other and the rest was easy. I had a lovely baby boy. He didn't cry and was blue around the lips so I blew down his mouth and up his nose (I don't know why!) and he gave a little cry. I shouted down to Charlie that we had a lovely son and can't describe how overjoyed I felt.

He dashed up to me with my niece and one of my neighbours and put a blanket around us. The ambulancemen came and checked us and the umbilical cord and said all was fine: then the midwife came. They carried me into the bedroom. The midwife congratulated me and said I'd done very well. I'd done the right thing to clear my baby's mucous. I didn't need any stitches but in my joy I'd forgotten the placenta. My baby, Lee John, weighed 5lb 6oz and was born at 1.39pm on 14th August. We had to go into the hospital as Lee was premature.

I loved the way I had my baby and wouldn't have wished it any other way. I held him straight from birth for five precious minutes or more, on my own. It was the best experience I have ever had in my whole life. My son will soon be nine years old. We are so close, and he is a very loving child.

SUSAN McCROSSAN

HELEN
AMMERLAAN

I didn't want to move to Gloucestershire. It wasn't that I'd anything against this county, I just didn't want to move. We'd only been back in Cheshire for a year with Nick commuting at weekends – which obviously wasn't ideal. We were all settled with our various activities and friends. We weren't exactly dragged kicking and screaming down the motorway, as the children missed their Daddy and I missed my husband, but suffice to say no-one (except Nick) looked forward wholeheartedly to the move.

We had made the most of our weekends together, as I was almost three months pregnant when we moved! Before leaving Cheshire, I'd obtained the number of my new NCT contact – a great network, the NCT – and had found out from her a doctor who was sympathetic to home confinements.

We moved in – I hated the house, hated the village – nothing was the same (obviously!); the NCT was organised slightly differently. The village seemed to be full of people over 50 – I knew no other pregnant women and it rained all the time. I don't even enjoy being pregnant – the only light at the end of the tunnel was that the babe was going to be born at home.

Slowly some things began to change; I did discover that there were some families with children in the village; I started to teach a set of classes, the women all due to deliver at about the same time as myself – so now I knew some other pregnant women. I might be an antenatal teacher but I had the same needs as any pregnant woman and I needed to discuss my pregnancy with others in the same situation. I didn't feel so isolated now – but still it rained!

We went North for a visit and it seemed noisy and crowded; things I thought I was missing I realised I no longer missed. We returned 'home' and the sun was shining.

I was convinced that I would go to my delivery date; in spite of telling classes to have an open mind about their baby's birth date, I had set ideas. I'd even convinced my midwife. However, babe had other ideas. The day I started in labour was not the most convenient of days. I had things planned, my husband had an early, important meeting, the midwife wasn't on duty and even the doctor had taken his car into the garage! It was also the last day of the summer holidays and I hadn't even discussed where the children would go in such an eventuality.

By 8.00am I was definitely in labour; a new friend who had lent me a wicker basket for the baby had offered to help out if I needed her, and happily for my children, hers were of the same age. Luckily she was up and collected my two just after the midwife arrived, at 8.30am.

I was on the bathroom floor when I met the midwife – I had this need to earth myself during a contraction. I was examined – five centimetres dilated – halfway there. Another midwife had gone off sick, so my regular lady was now on duty, so things were going well. The whole experience was lovely. At 10.49am the baby arrived quietly, calmly, no fuss; we discovered he was a boy. He quietly started to breathe, he was wide awake and alert and fed right away. I had opted for a physiological third stage and some 40 minutes later the placenta was delivered. Nick cut the cord and our baby was now a separate being. The sun was shining.

The sun stayed out for the rest of the week. My memories of that time are of calm and peacefulness and Jonathon on the whole reflects this. He is a very peaceful and calm babe.

I now like the house, how could I not, as our baby son was born there? When thinking about having a home confinement, and giving reasons for your choice to midwives, doctors and consultants, I don't really suppose this one counts very highly on their lists, but Jonathon's birth in this house has really made it into our home.

LESLEY
HOBBS

At 8.00am I notice irregular contractions. Definitely not Braxton Hicks, nor 'practice' contractions. I am excited, and ablaze with energy, my body burning to be active. I begin to organise and become increasingly 'busy'. The bedroom must be prepared – therefore I lift every stick of furniture about, washing everything – (and I *mean* everything) with Milton. I open the cupboards, wash mirrors, change sheets, vacuum the carpet. I know things are getting desperate when I find myself washing the outside of the windows! I get the delivery packs out, and put things tidily in readiness for the midwife – this is the first time I do this – I shall rearrange things at least five more times in the course of the day.

I get out various things for myself, keeping it all to a minimum; soap, towels, flannel and nightie for after the bath; mist spray (well, a plant spray and a bottle of mineral water) a bottle of fizzy apple juice and a teacher-beaker for during labour. I heap the bed with an enormous floor cushion and lots of pillows and put old sheets on it, on top of a big sheet of plastic. I prepare the cradle for the baby, and make sure that a soft flanelette sheet and clean soft clothes are readily accessible.

11.00am and I am still full of this feeling of energy; I must burn it off or explode, I feel. The contractions are still irregular – I announce my intention of going to the bank – my mother has trouble recovering from the shock of being driven to the shops by a woman in labour. On our return I tell the children I think the baby will come today. My three year old son is a bit upset; we had spent a long time talking about Mummy having 'our' baby at home, only to have our hard work undone by well-meaning but interfering women who say to him, 'Oh no, darling, babies are born in hospital!' I am enraged by this – a close friend of ours died recently in hospital, and my poor child is very apprehensive about Mummy's well-being. So, I laboriously explain, yet again, that we intend that the baby will be born in our house, in our bed, and hope it works. My 20-month old daughter doesn't give a damn, my dear, she never does about *anything* . . . oh, well, I phone the midwife. 'I think we're off,' I say. 'OK,' she says casually, 'You should know. I'll pop round.' All rather anticlimactic, really. I also phone my husband. He is, naturally, in a meeting. His secretary, an over-excitable girl, instantly becomes over-excited, so, lest anyone should think me over-excited, I promptly become off-hand and casual myself. Perhaps she could ask him to amble home at some point? Thank you so much, no not terribly wound-up, third time, you know, ha ha, yes, cheerio – and despise myself for my snobbery and unkindness in not sharing my good feelings with the poor girl – it's just that she gushes so . . .

I have been taking various homeopathic remedies to prevent me from being as copiously sick this time as I have been on my previous two labours: I hope they work. I mutter to myself as I down the last evil-smelling, putrid-tasting dose. My parents are very interested in the way things are done today; my mother was intrigued when I told her that people have to insist to get home deliveries now – she feels strongly that home is the right place for birth, as it is for most other things. I think she's right.

2.00pm. All my arrangements are made. The midwife has been – although she thinks it might all come to nothing, or be a long time because the cervix isn't effaced yet, I know I'm going to have this baby today. The energy surge is fading, the contractions are getting stronger and rather more regular. Pete is home, and I spend a lot of time holding his hand. I need his strength and his steadiness – I don't know how women survive emotionally, going through labour without their men. Tears come into my eyes at the thought, and he understands. I go up to my bedroom to catch a little sleep before things really begin to shift, but I can't sleep, so I rest instead. My mother comes and talks to me – I find her presence more than comforting. We laugh together, sharing experiences. It's good.

4.00pm. After a couple of hours, I wander downstairs for some tea to drink – I can hear cups chinking, and it makes me thirsty. The contractions have changed their nature – they are becoming much stronger now. I want to make sure that the children are settled before I go upstairs again. I don't want the kids around when the contractions get really heavy so I must tell them now that I shall go upstairs soon, and I won't be down again until the baby comes.

5.00pm. Time to go up. The midwife returns, I am 50 per cent effaced, but the os is so posterior, she can't find it. She has tiny hands and I have a posterior os – we've always had this problem! She trots off to grab some dinner and get 'the stuff' as she calls it – gas and air machine, and resuscitation kit: I know I shan't use the former, or need the latter, but she gets it anyway and ignores my conceit.

6.00pm. The contractions are beginning to really bite. I have forgotten – oh God, have I forgotten – just how much it hurts. My body is grabbed in a vice – I go rigid before a gentle touch on the nape of my neck reminds me to relax, breathe out, go with it, not against it. Again, I am obsessed by the fear that Pete will go away, disappear, vanish. I cling around his neck like a vine. Choking, he gently disengages himself and we giggle like a couple of nervous children. Whole chunks of minutes go by without me noticing. I feel safe here, something I hadn't felt in either previous labour – I am suddenly aware of that feeling of 'home-ness', of familiarity and warmth. That's another plus to chalk up for home deliveries.

7.00pm. Another vaginal examination and the cervix is fully effaced but not dilated. I am fully in the grip of labour now, and everything slides past, looking and sounding like a dream. The only real thing is me and what's happening to me. In a dream I clutch at Pete, in a dream the midwife tells me I'm not dilating yet. I am, however, vomiting, which ranks as one of life's nastier and unmistakeable realities. My friend had her baby this morning. It took two hours, according to her abominably smug husband. Every so often, this fact returns to me and I am heard to mutter furiously, 'Two hours! Expletive deleted, two hours!' I am given apple juice to drink, in case I become dehydrated with all this vomiting. It's lovely, and so refreshing: so is the water spray.

8.00pm. Still not dilating – in the midst of my dream, I become anxious. I have fears of being taken to hospital, and all that entails. The vomiting, thank goodness, has stopped.

8.45pm. Midwife wants to do another examination. I swear at her, furiously afraid that I am not dilating, knowing that I want to push, and only too well aware of the effects of pushing on a closed cervix. I tell her to leave me alone, only to be over-ruled by Pete who calmly tells her to go ahead – he will deal with me – I am outraged, but know he is right. The midwife realises that my extremely tough membranes are actually holding the cervix almost shut; she struggles with her tiny hands, and an amnio-hook and – oh, the relief! A jet of water shoots out under pressure, and I actually feel my cervix dilate like a burst balloon. I am up on my knees, a position I have found more comfortable for the last couple of hours, and I feel the baby move down. The delight and relief are immeasurable.

9.00pm and I push! Oh boy, do I push. I push again, shouting in triumph as the baby's head emerges – then remember, guiltily, everyone else in the house. I am reassured – they are all at the other end of the house and can't hear me. I'd hate to frighten the kids now it's all nearly over! A wriggle, a slither and another beautiful, wonderful miracle of a daughter lands squalling on the bed. It's 9.15pm.

The cord is cut, it's stopped pulsating. I feed my Susannah, and we croon nonsense to her as the doctor and midwife grin happily. The placenta comes out, it's tea-time, I've deserved it – but those heroes around me have really earned it!

I was recently privileged to be with two of my closest friends when their son, Nikhil, was born. Sharon has two other children whose labours were both difficult, painful and frightening. For this labour she wanted to be more in touch with the processes her body was working through and – like most of us – she wanted to stay as comfortable as possible! She and Girish were very attracted by the idea of a water birth at home as this seemed to offer all the qualities they required for both mother and baby. Reports of water birth suggested that the water not only provided a gentle transition for the baby from its enclosed uterine world to the new and open environment of our world; but also that the mother's pain was relieved by the warmth and support of the water.

Technical information was obtained from a number of sources and various publications. Eventually, after some sifting of the details, a very simple procedure became clear:

1) Don't get in too early (pre-five centimetres dilation) as this seems to slow early labour (too relaxing?).

2) It is not necessary to add salt to the water.

3) Ordinary tap water is just fine.

4) The temperature needs to be kept at between 98°F and 100°F. Birthing tubs you can hire have a built in heater which controls this thermostatically. We actually raised the water temperature to 101°F just prior to the birth so Nikhil was welcomed into a really warm environment. Some studies suggest you should drop the water temperature by a few degrees in second stage to help the expulsive contractions.

5) A baby doesn't need to breathe unaided until the cord pulsing has slowed to a level where the baby is no longer receiving sufficient oxygen from its mother. Its first breath is usually stimulated by previously empty (of gas) airways meeting our atmosphere which rushes in to fill it up and so inflates the lungs. So if the airways don't feel air, that response does not occur. It takes a lot of confidence to keep a newborn baby under the water even if you believe this and most midwives I have met are not willing to leave the baby underwater for more than a few seconds. Another objection often raised at this point is that even if air cannot and does not need to be breathed in at this time, there will continue to be fluid exchange, just as the baby in utero 'breathes' amniotic fluid in and out.

The water in a birthing tub may well be pretty murky by this time and there is some concern that the baby may inspire or ingest impure water. These questions cannot really be answered until more research has been done. Consequently many women

SHEILA KEAN

choose to labour in water and get out for delivery.

Sharon and Girish chose to hire a fish pond for their labour. It was an ideal height for Girish, the midwives and me to attend to Sharon; its contours provided useful platforms to sit on, kneel against or lean on and it was deep enough in the middle for Sharon to lie completely immersed. It was filled by a hosepipe from the hot tap and emptied by siphoning using the same hosepipe, we kept the temperature constant by adding sauce-panfuls of hot water. It really wasn't an arduous task but it does need a third party to enable the woman to receive constant support.

Sharon started contracting at about 2.00am on Friday morning and I joined them at about 4.00am. The next 15 hours passed in a haze of preparing and eating food (have to keep the strength up after all); a freezing cold walk (supposedly to stimulate contractions but I'm sure the adverse weather made us all so uncomfortable it had the opposite effect); and a few hours rest. During this time contractions were coming every ten minutes and lasting 90 seconds or so and Sharon was working beautifully with these by entering a very quiet and peaceful state and breathing deeply and gently. By about 8.00pm on Friday Nikhil, who had been in a posterior position, had turned and the cervix began to dilate. The contractions became much more insistent and Sharon was using light, swift breathing to stay on top of them. She continued to use this throughout the rest of labour, combining it with counting and loving eye-contact from Girish.

A visit from Sister J. confirmed Sharon was two and a half centimetres dilated and she left expecting to visit us on Saturday morning. Sharon got into a hot bath at this point which made the pain more bearable. She stayed there for one and a half hours, either reclining or on all fours, while Girish counted and I poured water on to her from a jug. Eventually the bath became too confining and the pond was prepared. It was wonderful to watch Sharon slide into it and just unfold. She was able to change position easily – reclining, floating, kneeling, squatting, sitting – and was 'buoyed up' by the water in more ways than one. Time passed quickly and peacefully and it was exhilarating to watch Sharon respond to the sensations within her body and also to watch Girish responding to her needs and feeding her the love and strength she needed through his looks and touch.

At 1.00am on Saturday morning Sharon was starting to show signs of transition – shivering, grunting and feeling sick – so she got out of the tub for a while until the water was brought up to 101°F. Towels, nappies and a little nightie were placed on the radiator to warm. The midwife was called and she and her student arrived about 1.15am. Vaginal examination revealed that the cervix was eight centimetres dilated and Sharon thankfully returned to the tub.

Once back in the tub the contractions came fast and furious and Sharon 'got on with it'. It was an amazing experience to watch the real power of woman as she prepared to release her child into the world outside her body. The midwives were wonderful – just sitting back and letting it all happen, but providing a marvellous sense of security and support. As the time for Nikhil's birth approached Sharon was encouraged to adopt a squatting/ kneeling forwards posture, leaning on the edge of the pool. Nikhil's head was delivered very slowly (no tearing despite large episiotomies on both previous occasions), and must have remained under water for about 60–90 seconds before the rest of his body emerged and he was lifted up out of the water. He was 'posted' through Sharon's legs and after she had settled back down into the water she took Nikhil into her arms and held him in the water, with just his head out, while he fed and looked around with those all-knowing newborn eyes. It was 2.35am. Unlike most newborns he never did curl back into a foetal position and clench his fists. His arms seemed to be spread wide open in a joyful embrace of his new world.

The placenta was delivered naturally about 30 minutes after the birth and within an hour the new family were tucked up in bed eating Nikhil's birthday cake. By 4.30am the tub was emptied, the washing on and we were all peacefully asleep.

I shall never be able to thank Sharon, Girish and Nikhil enough for letting me share that very special and miraculous time. I would also like to thank the midwives not only for making me feel so welcome and useful but for restoring my faith in what midwifery can and should be like.

SHARON PATEL

When I thought I might be pregnant (but rather doubted it), I took some urine to the Health Centre for a pregnancy test. Imagine my surprise when the test was done on the spot! A few minutes later, with, 'Yes, you're definitely pregnant,' ringing in my ears, I found myself being asked by the booking clerk, pen poised, 'Which hospital do you want to have your baby in?' A small clear voice rose from within me: 'I am going to have a home birth'.

At just a few weeks from conception, my child within clearly told me what kind of birth he wanted. We attended a seminar on water births, read books on the subject, meditated and practised yoga. Our whole life-style is aimed at living as close to nature as possible and Girish and I had total faith that the pregnancy and birth would be perfect in accordance with Nature's plan.

We very much wanted a gentle birth. It was as important to us that our baby's transition from the womb was as gentle and trauma free as that I was comfortable during labour. The soothing and healing properties of water would therefore help me and my baby, and our ideas of a water birth changed into definite plans and preparations.

I felt that the smooth, contoured pool we were given by the aquatic centre was perfect. We had a few 'trial runs' to test the speed of filling the pool and to check that we could maintain the water temperature at 101°F. I could then test the pool for comfort and ease of acquiring different positions.

As the birth drew near, I prepared the room by keeping fresh flowers in it (an abundance of daffodils); and placing inspiring pictures around. There was a beautiful large candle we were to light when labour began. The pool was in the centre of the room so that there was access to me from every angle.

My birth attendants were to be my husband, Girish, my friend Sheila Kean and Sister J. with a student midwife. We got to know Sister J. before the birth and appreciated her reassuring manner and her willingness to assist us in our chosen method of birth. Sheila gave me a weekly massage up to the birth so we felt connected and prepared in our own ways.

As it turned out, my labour lasted for about twenty-five hours. I hadn't anticipated that my baby would be in a posterior positon and that it would take so long to rotate into the correct position. Sheila joined us in the early hours of the morning and soon after arriving was cooking vast pots of soup and making huge amounts of apple crumble and the like. The kitchen became full to bursting with food which, amazingly, we managed to get through by the end of the day!

The first part of my labour was very gentle and we talked, dozed, ate, and even went for a short walk in the woods; but later in the evening it became more intense as I began to dilate. When the contractions became very strong I got in the bath and felt the water as immediate relief. Sheila poured water over my back while Girish prepared the pool.

By the time I got into the pool, the contractions were coming almost without a break. Girish maintained eye contact with me all the time and looked so calm and loving as we breathed and counted through the contractions together. I remember him telling me that I looked beautiful, I was so thankful that with all my yoga practice I could relax my body during the contractions and noted how the pain increased if for a split second panic set in.

Sister J. arrived for the last hour. I appreciated her calm, gentle manner and was hardly aware of her presence. I was leaning forward over the edge of the pond and as far as I was concerned only Girish and Sheila were there. Sister J. and the student were behind me.

During the second stage I found that I could control the speed of the birth, and rather than pushing, I let my body do most of the work, and found that the deep throaty noise I made released my tensions. I felt Nikhil being born gently into the water and I saw tears rolling down Girish's cheeks. It seemed to me that at the moment of birth time stood still and there was total silence that was quite magical.

When I first saw and held our son he looked so quiet and peaceful, just looking around, and I felt he was the most beautiful being I'd ever seen. I was, and still am, over-awed by his beauty and welcome the immense privilege of being his mother.

I know that every birth is unique and wonderful and I can speak only from my own experience (having had two hospital births), that a gentle birth at home (especially in water) has everything to commend it. It was a natural process rather than an organized one and I was free to do whatever I liked in my own familiar surroundings. It was wonderful just to be with Girish and Sheila who were so calm and loving. I definitely recommend having a close friend with you as well as your husband for a home birth.

I can say without question that water is beneficial for both mother and baby, and I was so relieved not to have torn (having had two previous episiotomies). I feel that one of the greatest joys of this birth experience was to be left alone, just the three of us — simply to go upstairs, sharing the wonder of it all, and then blissful sleep!

SUSAN
JONES

On my first visit to antenatal clinic I was duly booked into hospital, etc., etc. I think I said yes to all these things as I was still in a state of shock at being pregnant. However, having time to think about it, I returned a month later determined to have a home birth, preferably water if possible. I found little initial resistance from either the midwives or the doctors at the surgery. However, later the doctors, realising I was serious, objected and struck me out of their care (although this was due to insurance purposes and they were always there if I needed them and would have come to the birth if needed).

The midwives, however, from start to finish were brilliant, although daunted at the prospect and a little nervous. They fully supported me and were very sympathetic to my wishes for a natural pregnancy and birth. In fact, the only upsetting time I had during my pregnancy was being sent to see a consultant at the local hospital – which was a horrible experience and was the cause of feeling unwell for a few days afterwards. I felt insignificant, foolish, guilty, doubtful and most of all my confidence was temporarily taken away, as were feelings of power over my own feelings and body – to think that some women submit themselves to this kind of attitude at such a wonderful time in their lives is truly saddening.

I must point out here that from the beginning I felt absolutely healthy and well and I felt that my baby was also healthy and well – had I felt that at any time there was any doubt, I would not have hesitated in seeking medical advice; likewise, if I had felt that the birth would be difficult. I would have gone into hospital – after all, it is the baby's life that is of the utmost importance. Anyway, I decided not to have a scan, as I felt no need. This wasn't very well received either. I made sure I ate well during my pregnancy. The only supplement to my diet was Floradix, a herbal iron tonic, containing many natural sources of vitamins and minerals, as I am allergic to iron tablets.

I privately arranged the hire of my watertub and went to collect it two weeks before my expected date with my father. We then had a practice run, which was just as well as we found a problem with the water supply which I then got repaired. Actually, the practice was a bit of a shambles but we all decided that this was a good omen! I practised on my own later with more success. One factor which had been a slight worry to the doctors was that I lived 20 miles from the hospital in a remote farmhouse, but as I was happy with the arrangements that fact faded into the background and the midwives loved coming to see me at home.

During my pregnancy I regularly had shiatsu, which helped to keep me physically well – I had been told by an osteopath when I was younger that if ever I got pregnant I would have big trouble with my back, but I was not affected any more than usual by backache. I also had a number of re-birthing sessions which helped me emotionally and I gave myself Reiki which I practice anyway. Actually, I had never felt healthier or happier. The night before my due date I felt odd, my dog noticing this first. I tried to sleep and couldn't so woke my mother and told her I thought I had food poisoning. So we carefully began filling the tub, I got in and out at various stages and telephoned the midwife early in the morning, who came out and told me that my labour hadn't properly started yet and went off to do her clinic and would be back later. It was a midwife I was particularly friendly with, which added to my pleasure. Having my mother there as my only attendant was brilliant and has brought us even closer, and being at home felt so good.

Later that day, much earlier than expected, things really began to happen. I used breathing techniques to control the pain and contractions (I did have a puff of gas and air but felt it interfered with my job). The midwife had brought a student with her whom I also knew and liked – this was because they had been doing clinic together and came straight afterwards. It was nice to see them relaxed, laughing and talking around me in my own home.

Just after 3.30pm I gave birth very easily to a lovely baby daughter Shoshanna who stayed under water for a couple of minutes. She was so calm and relaxed it was amazing and already had her eyes open under the water. We placed her on my chest and she just looked at me for ages as if to say, 'so that's what you look like'.

I think everyone agreed that the waterbirth was a very good way to have a baby. I had her in the squatting position which I naturally took up; on dry land that may have been more difficult. I know I certainly benefited from the water, and so did Shoshanna – a safe, familiar medium midway between womb and air to allow her to adjust more gently. As I lay exhausted on my mattress, I thought numerous times how grateful I was to be in the peace and quiet of my own home, which made the whole experience so much more special. It was also nice to receive my very supportive family and friends and to show them where it all happened afterwards. My Mum thought it was very special too and said how privileged she felt to have been there playing such an important role in the birth of her grand daughter.

See pictures page 130

KAREN HIBBS

I was beginning to think labour would never start because after a tummy upset at 31–32 weeks resulting in contractions and admission to hospital, I had 'niggled' all the time, forever thinking 'is this it?' It was a relief when we collected the birthing pool; I was getting worried that my water birth wouldn't happen.

On the morning of 6th July (one week overdue) I woke with a jump at 2.00am to the sensation of a small leak of warm water. I was initially excited, then wary that it might just be an embarrassment! So, I went back to sleep and woke again at 8.00am with the same thing, only this time I was pretty certain, as despite pulling up my pelvic floor, water continued to leak. Whilst getting myself and my two sons dressed I had a few mild contractions which continued all day.

My midwife came at about 9.30am and when she did an internal she said the forewaters were intact (the membrane in front of the baby's head) but could tell that there was liquor draining, so drew the conclusion that I had had a hindwater rupture (a hole at the top of the bag of membranes). The cervix was three centimetres dilated, a great joy for me because a week before, despite eight weeks of niggles, the cervix was tightly closed.

So, I was on my way at last. I was really excited but as the morning wore on I began to get nervous – I can cope with first stage but I always dread second stage. I almost phoned my husband to ask him to come home but by keeping myself busy I managed to keep fairly calm. I washed, tidied and cleaned so that my husband would have little to do for a couple of days. I took my eldest to playgroup which was my downfall – the teachers and another pregnant mum were all excited for me and it got my adrenalin and nerves going. Back at home with the younger one in bed I was alone and shaking like a leaf. Action again saved the day; I began to prepare my delivery room. A tray with cups, coffee, tea, etc., moving chairs and tables into better positions and finally putting water into the pool. It was already one third full with cold water which we had done a couple of days earlier, and it was now time to start and warm it up. The cylinder of hot water filled it to about two thirds the level I would need and a bit hotter than the desired 36–37 degrees which would gradually cool and leave us with only a small top up to do later. (We had kept a cylinder full of very hot water for a week in readiness for filling the pool).

I found it quite relaxing, just sitting in my chosen room watching the water level gradually rise; it was very tempting to get in.

My midwife came back at 2.30pm and although contractions were only mild I had dilated to four centimetres.

My Dad did playgroup duty and then took the boys off to his house armed with all the necessaries for an overnight stay.

When Nick came home at 4.30pm we didn't know what to do with ourselves; it was so quiet without the boys. We forced a bit of tea down (neither of us had an appetite), then we finished filling the pool.

The midwife returned at 6.30pm to re-assess the situation. There was slight progress, the cervix now four centimetres plus dilated and the head had come down. During an internal the forewaters broke; the towels, etc., that we had put on the bed only just coped with the seemingly endless flow of warm water.

Over the next couple of hours contractions gradually increased in frequency and strength. Although I could cope well with them I was fidgety and didn't want to sit down, so while the midwife and my husband drank coffee and chatted I was out in the garden getting the dry washing in and folding it; 'the things these women do', as the midwife said. But if I didn't do it then, when was Nick going to get a chance to do it? By 9.00 pm, we decided it was probably OK to get into the pool as contractions were now about every two to three minutes and fairly strong, but to check progress the midwife did an internal. Just as the books recommend for entering the pool, I was five centimetres dilated. I was a little nervous – what if it wasn't what I hoped; what if it didn't work at all?

I soon discovered my fears were unfounded; the warm water was heaven. I knelt, leaning my forearms along the edge of the pool. Nick pulled up a stool and had one arm around my shoulders while I gripped the other one. The water was very relaxing, enabling me to rest well between contractions. Once I was in the water, things really speeded up. The contractions seemed to come a lot closer together and were a lot stronger.

My mind was in two distinct halves – one swearing away to itself about how awful it was, the other revelling in the pleasure of being in the beautiful warm water. Everything was very peaceful, just the quiet voices of Nick and the midwife giving encouragement. Despite the strong contractions and the pain and discomfort caused by them I was wonderfully relaxed, more so than when I was on dry land and contracting less strongly.

Presumably because of my relaxed state, labour progressed rapidly. Within half an hour of entering the pool I had an urge to push, and 10 minutes later at 10.00pm, my baby was born. I had moved round so that the midwife could guide the head out but I stayed in the same position. The birth took place under the water and the baby just floated to the top, spine uppermost, head, arms and legs hanging weightless. I gently put my hand under the baby's chest and pulled the baby up and back until it was leaning on my chest and the first breath of life quietly happened; no loud noises, no sudden movements. It was beautiful. Then we had to untangle, or so it seemed, the legs and umbilical cord to identify the baby's sex – another boy, Gareth Edward, who weighed in at 8lb 8oz. He suffered absolutely no after effects of being delivered under the water and is a beautiful, fit and healthy little boy.

Prior to labour, the midwife had asked me if I wanted Syntometrine for the third stage of labour. As I couldn't come to any real decision she decided to leave it ready in the syringe just in case we needed it. I stayed in the water and after about 10 minutes I pushed the placenta out.

Then I climbed out of the pool and was amazed when I stood up at how heavy my stomach felt; I knew that being in water makes you feel weightless, but I had not realised until that moment. I did not need any stitches, another advantage of being in water apparently. Then I had a bath and sat cuddling my new baby.

The pool was well worth every penny we spent on the hire charge. I certainly recommend the use of water in labour and will definitely have a pool again for my next labour. Many people at work asked why I didn't use the ordinary bath and before labour I knew it wouldn't be effective; now I know there is just no comparison. I had put two large blankets on the floor of the pool underneath the liners and these were nice and soft to tread on. We had no bright lights in the room; the whole atmosphere was calm and relaxed. I feel very lucky to have been able to have my baby at home but I also had the wonderful bonus of a waterbirth. I had an open mind before labour about delivery in the water; primarily, I wanted the water for relaxation and pain relief. It certainly relaxed me; I'm not sure how much pain relief there was. My overriding feeling was for safety. If at any stage it was felt by anybody that it would be best to leave the pool then I would have done so.

See picture page 59

TWINS AND TRIPLETS

Parents of twins often expect the birth to be difficult, but our reports show that this is not necessarily the case. We have a quick and straightforward delivery, a premature birth, a forceps delivery and even triplets born by Caesarean. Multiple pregnancies may present extra challenges, but the reports illustrated show how the parents came to terms with these and indeed found extra joy in having more than one baby.

MARTINE ARCHER

I had twins and went through a lot of upset which all turned out to be for nothing. When I initially discussed with my Consultant about wanting a natural labour and delivery, he sat and listened and then said, 'well, we like all twin deliveries to have an epidural' and went on to describe internal manipulation of the second twin, how painful it could be and the high risk of death or damage with twin births. I went on to see the Senior Midwife as he had quite upset me. Her only comment was I should be grateful he wasn't insisting on a Caesarean and that anything should be endured to have a live healthy baby. She also told me that epidurals did not add to the risk of an assisted delivery, which is a blatant lie.

I went through several weeks of reading up, talking to people and feeling tense about the whole prospect before I decided the risk to myself and the babies was worse with the epidural and told the Consultant I wouldn't have one. I felt so much better once I had made my decision and felt confident in my ability to cope with the birth of my twins, especially after they had both settled head down.

In the end all the upset was unnecessary since I only had a two hour labour, reached hospital fully dilated and was delivered by the midwife naturally with only a small cut. The main point I really want to make is that nobody went out of their way to explain the problems of epidurals; I only learned about them by reading widely. I feel that a lot of women with twins are probably pressurised unnecessarily into epidurals and all the ensuing problems with assisted delivery, drugged babies, possible lumbar puncture, blood pressure dropping, etc. I was made to feel that I didn't have the babies' interests at heart and I was being very selfish wanting any kind of decent birth experience (I had a very bad one with my first child). Without exception, all the twin mums I have spoken to had either Caesarean or assisted delivery for either or both twins, and I was concerned to support or give example to women wanting something more normal. It is possible!

See picture page 132

At thirty weeks pregnant with twins I was feeling big, a little tired but well after a few months respite from morning sickness and heartburn.

Waking up in the early hours of the morning as usual I tripped to the loo; I was shocked and a little shaky when I realised that I had most likely had a slight show. I woke my husband Brian and we decided I should telephone the hospital. The nurse suggested that if I was worried I should come to the hospital to check things were alright, especially as I was having twins. I very much needed this reassurance; therefore, after packing a bag just in case I was admitted for a day or so, we anxiously set off to hospital.

After various nurses had a good press on my tummy to feel the babies' positions (this was quite uncomfortable), monitors were fitted to record their heart rates – all was well. A young, sleepy doctor examined me (I recall asking if an internal examination could start off labour and was told not). It was decided, because I was pregnant with twins, that I should be admitted for observation. Brian then went home to prepare for a normal day at work.

At about 8.00am I went to the loo; this time I was losing blood. Obviously extremely concerned, I told the couple of nurses who, rather uncaringly, I thought, said that I'd only had 'a show' and was told to go back to bed, so I did. At this point my waters broke, which started the beginning of premature labour. I cried for the first time and felt very frightened and alone. I asked if anything could be done to stop my labour; I was told no. I felt that I badly needed lots of calm, positive reassurances that my babies would be alright, but no-one talked to me about what premature labour would mean and I was given no information. An auxiliary nurse tried to comfort me by putting an arm around my shoulder, but I interpreted this as sympathy which worried me even more and made me more upset. I think she was a little bemused that I rejected her.

When Brian returned to the hospital I had been transferred to the labour ward. It made such an enormous difference to have him with me – the shock of it all had made us both silly and I remember we laughed a lot and made jokes (needless to say my contractions were not too painful at this stage). We made a final decision on what to call the babies, after the deliberations and name combinations over the months. At no time did we speak of fears that the babies could die – our concerns couldn't stretch beyond that they would be born as healthy as possible in view of their prematurity.

The monitors were fitted again; eventually, I asked for them to be removed as they were so uncomfortable. I was also

SUE
RICHARDS

catheterised for a short while. The pain relief I was offered was gas and air – this I found very useful as I tried to focus on the method of using it (which fortunately I had just been taught how to do by my NCT teacher at antenatal classes) in order to try to block out the pain of the contractions. After a short first stage of about four hours I felt the sensation to push. I recall thinking whether I did want to push or was it my imagination? The feeling came again and I asked Brian to tell the nurse. As a result of Brian being with me and his natural, calm way of helping me, I felt fairly good at this stage, as though some 'normality' had returned and I was not over-anxious – in fact I was rather pleased with myself that I had recognised this mystical urge to push I'd read about, although Brian had apparently gone out of the room and told the nurse that I 'felt funny!'

I was fully dilated and about to give birth so was rushed to the delivery room – without my gas and air or Brian who was quickly informed that he couldn't be present in the delivery room in case of complications (this was a relief to him as he had always felt that he preferred not to be at the birth unless I felt that I needed him there).

The delivery room was busy with two midwives, two doctors to deliver the babies, two paediatricians and a nurse and an onlooker. I hadn't yet reached antenatal classes regarding 'pushing' and this, as well as a fear of somehow hurting the babies, I found confusing – also after a few pushes with midwives holding my legs, my feet were put in stirrups which I was not happy with. I was told that an episiotomy would be done to protect the babies heads and ease the delivery.

It was perhaps 15 minutes before our daughter was born. I didn't see her or hear her but was told the baby was a girl and did we have a name for her? The waters of the second twin were broken by the doctor and immediately I had two contractions and two minutes later our son was born. Again I didn't see him; I remember feeling surprised when I heard a baby's cry (I must have thought they'd alredy been taken to SCBU). I was stunned that everything seemed to have happened so quickly. I owe thanks to the student midwife who thoughtfully put her hand out to momentarily stop the incubator which was rushing our daughter out of the delivery room; she gave me my first brief, precious sight of my baby. The paediatrician had a quick word as he left with the babies: he kindly said that he would visit me on the ward later to let me know how they were.

Although our son, the second twin, was lying transverse, he simply followed the lead of his sister and both babies were quickly born head first without the need for forceps. However, a most distressing time occurred when I was being stitched. I hadn't been given enough local anaesthetic and was feeling every tug and pull as the stitches went in – I called out in pain and the same pupil midwife drew the fact to the attention of the doctor performing the task.

Shortly after the birth Brian came into the delivery room; we were given two polaroid photos of the babies and spent some time there together; we were both quite 'high' and so very pleased that we had two beautiful babies. Brian went to SCBU and I was 'cleaned up' and transferred to the post-natal ward. He then left to see the new grandparents.

I feel my labour and delivery were treated very impersonally by the staff involved, except for the pupil midwife. I am sure that the experience would have been much less traumatic afterwards had this not been so. I am also left with a conflict of feelings however as obviously I am so grateful to the staff for the safe delivery of my babies. By this time the shock was beginning to increase and I tried hard to 'keep hold', trying to concentrate on practicalities such as which ward I was on, when visiting and meal times were. I was informed I had to stay in bed for six hours after which time I could visit my babies in intensive care. When the waiting was almost finished a nurse told me that because I had had twins I must stay in bed for 10 hours not six hours, and that I wouldn't be able to visit the SCBU until later. At that point I was unable to stop the floods of tears. I was so very disappointed and desperate, but in a shocked state of mind I was not strong enough to express my wishes and insist.

My reaction on seeing them for the first time was very confused – I was so sad that they looked so small and frail and seemed to me that they must be in pain and discomfort with drips and wires attached. I was frightened when the alarms sounded which made the nurses rush to check the babies were breathing (neither needed to be ventilated), the tears would not go away, nor would that dreadful uncertainty of whether or not they would come through all this. The Night Sister was very kind, patiently explaining how each twin was and the treatment they were having.

The babies very gradually progressed; they had some setbacks in the early days but no serious problems developed other than those which were expected with babies of their gestation. For Brian and me it was a very long, tiring nine weeks' wait, our emotions were so up and down, and at times, very much in the hands of the SCBU staff – a thoughtless remark could have a bad effect on our morale, but we were never in doubt of the loving care, skill and dedication the SCBU staff gave our babies.

One particular upset occurred when it was suggested we might take our son home first as he was feeding well and ready for discharge, leaving our daughter for a week or so until she gained more weight and was feeding better. I had left them both for so many weeks and felt I could not cope with leaving one of the babies behind – no they must both come home together if at all possible. It was agreed that both should stay for a little longer.

Before we brought the babies home I stayed for two days and two nights with them in the mother and baby room at the hospital. This was exhausting, as mothers were left to care for their babies with the staff being on hand to give advice if necessary. These two days of intensive motherhood were my making, giving me the confidence I badly needed to feel I could care for two premature babies at home.

This report is actually an extract from a letter written by the mother, who had conceived in Papua New Guinea, given birth in Zimbabwe and was writing to the father (Steve), who was touring Australia, had got as far as Tasmania, and had planned to be with his wife in time for the birth – only the twins arrived over six weeks early!

Sunday 3rd May

Lovely day with the family, large tea and a walk around the block – even for me! At 7.00pm I told sister Gerry that I thought the head had engaged. I (unusually for me) stayed up late hammering studs into a baby romper.

Twelve midnight – woken up by urge to wee. Got back into bed and immediately started uncontrollable wetting. Oh dear! Panic – call Gerry, who said whatever happens go to the hospital to confirm that the waters have broken and have a check up. Checked by midwife (four centimetres dilated). It took three sisters to find both heartbeats (and one was still convinced that there were three heads!)

1.30am and Mr. Gulliver came to check – set up a drip 'to control events' – a steroid injection to help develop the baby's lungs. Fortunately, I refused Ativan, (similar to Valium, and I knew it would make me sleep) which I think he offered because he thought I'd be in labour all day!

3.00am. Gerry was called back as contractions were coming every two minutes, but the sister said I was not just good, but 'excellent'! – doing all the right breathing exercises and not uttering a squeak. I puffed away until 5.00am, but kept wanting to open my bowels. The sister was a little concerned that I was confusing the sensation of wanting to push, and since I wasn't fully dilated she was afraid I would tear – apart from the fear of me popping a baby in the loo! At the next check the sister said my bladder was full, so we ventured forth to the loo, and I emptied myself thoroughly – felt much relieved and, having made the effort to get up, I was shunted straight back into the delivery ward as I was nine centimetres dilated at the last check. By the time I had returned, I was ready to push. Doc was called for action stations. It must have been soon after 5.00am. Sister said if possible not to push until the Gynae arrived. Fortunately he arrived quickly so I could start pushing, which I did for 35 minutes, before he performed an episiotomy and forceps delivery for Twin one. Nineteen minutes later Twin two arrived, after being turned from a transverse position by Mr Gulliver. Seemed like I was stitched up for hours! – but not too stiff or painful next day.

Notes from Mother

1) The news that I was carrying twins was broken in a psychologically positive way, in that it was early (11 weeks) by a British ex-pat Doctor who congratulated me and was very supportive and encouraging. Steve was like a cat who had got the cream throughout.

2) We had an excellent antenatal course which included a talk by the 'Susu-Mamas', and the breast feeding counsellor lent me leaflets on feeding twins – a complication it is easy to overlook!

3) I had a peaceful, restful three to four months – sewing, swimming, sleeping and eating 'by the book' – after the initial three months when I worked as a locum in a hospital and felt nauseous.

4) It was wonderful to be surrounded by my supportive family, with its laughing and excitement during the final month.

5) The twins were in incubators for the first four days, just to be sure, and to be kept separate from full term infants.

6) For the final stage, I was on my back with my legs strapped into stirrups, which I think in retrospect was probably what delayed Twin one's descent.

7) Despite not seeing or touching the babies until 10 hours after they were born, I had no difficulty bonding with them both equally, and at first sight experienced an overwhelming protective feeling.

At 33 weeks I didn't seem to be so very large, considering that at 22 weeks I was the size of somebody at full term. But then, after all, I was having triplets – as much of a surprise to me at my 17-week scan as to everybody else.

SARAH
MARSHALL

At 31 weeks I only completed half of my last day at work – I wasn't feeling too grand – rather tired in fact, so the hospital suggested that it might be quite a good idea if I were to go in to see them 'with my bag'.

In hospital, the Consultant explained to me that in my stomach were three little risks and, to put it into perspective, it wasn't a foregone conclusion that there would be three babies at the end of the day, but that he and the full paediatric teams were going to 'do their damndest'. After 10 days in hospital, only able to eat half a pot of yoghurt at a time because my stomach was so squashed, the consultant decided that as I had developed pre-eclampsia, I should have an elective Caesarean under general anaesthetic.

This was a decision that I have come to regret, and now, looking back, I wish I had challenged it. I knew from experience that I reacted badly to general anaesthetic, and I explained this to the appropriate people, but for some reason it was ignored. At the time I was told that having an epidural might not be such a good idea as the delivery room would be packed with all these paediatric teams urgently rushing around with three seven-week premature babies, and the fraught situation might upset me too much – I think they saw it as having one less problem to deal with, but I felt so vulnerable and hadn't even spoken to anyone who had produced triplets before, so I was prepared to take the doctors advice and do just as I was told.

In the anaesthetic room outside the operating/delivery room, the sister on my ward at the time bore witness to the song and dance that went on as the anaesthetists tried to 'put me under'. After prodding around in one arm unsuccessfully, they changed to the other arm. When no vein was forthcoming, they went back to the first arm. At this point I asked the sister who the man was in the brown suit coming at me with a bicycle pump with a needle at the end! Obviously my mind was playing games. Soon after the event I was to develop phlebitis, an inflammation of the veins, in my twice attacked arm.

When I came around from the anaesthetic I was greeted by the houseman who told me that I had two girls and a boy and all was well. The nurses gave me polaroid photos of the babies when they were moments old – a common practice in situations where the mother is not well enough to see her baby, or the new-born needs to go straight to SCBU.

The effects of the anaesthetic took over again and I slept until 5.30am the next morning when the sister, who had been nothing but good to me during my two week stay, came and asked me if I had seen my babies yet. Finding that I hadn't, she wheeled me straight to SCBU where I saw the children – two boys and a girl, not the two girls and a boy I had been told about! Still suffering from the after effects of the anaesthetic, I didn't want to hold my babies. I wanted to be able to remember the moment, and I wasn't at all sure I would be able to, I felt so light-headed. How I wish I had had the epidural. However, I did hold the little hands and stroke the faces through the incubator port-holes. They were seven weeks early and weighed $3^3/_4$lbs each, but I was lucky in that they were all very healthy and only stayed in the incubators for 24 hours as a precaution. Two of them had drips in their arms, and the other through his navel. They seemed very long and thin with suntans, although they weren't jaundiced. They slept on special alarm pads designed to trip if their breathing stopped, but somehow I had little or no fear for their survival.

The sister then took me back to the ward and helped me shower, insisting that we then go straight back to SCBU. I think she was rather surprised and concerned about my attitude, but I knew how I felt, and, returning to SCBU, I was ready. I held one baby, I held another, I held the other. I held two together, I held all three together, I smiled! What was in store? I knew no-one could tell me.

Over the next few days I dragged myself down to SCBU. Those who have had a Caesarean will understand what it is like to roll onto your side on the bed before you drop off onto your hands and knees because you haven't got the muscles to pull yourself up into a sitting position, and how you have to start walking almost bent double, using door handles and tables to gradually pull yourself upright, and to shuffle along with your knees fixed so that you won't jar this stitched up blancmange that you are sure belongs to someone else.

Anyway, most of my waking, shuffling hours were spent in SCBU, bottle feeding, changing nappies, breastfeeding, changing nappies, bathing little bodies, changing nappies – I remember thinking that if I had a penny for every nappy I was going to have to change over the duration . . . but those babies could have been anybody's, I was just going through the motions of being a mother. It wasn't until the Thursday, six days after they were born, that I walked into SCBU early one morning when all was unusually calm, and something surged inside me, I had a lump in my throat and my stomach flipped – at last they felt mine and I

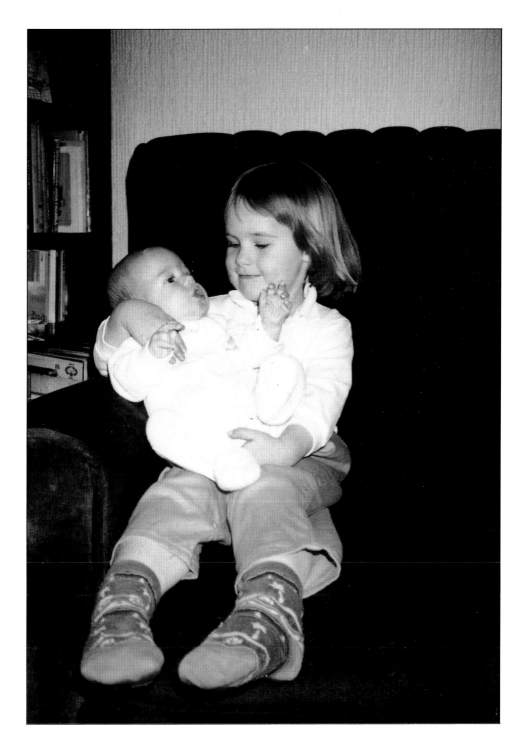

Kathy Aitchison with new baby brother Mike

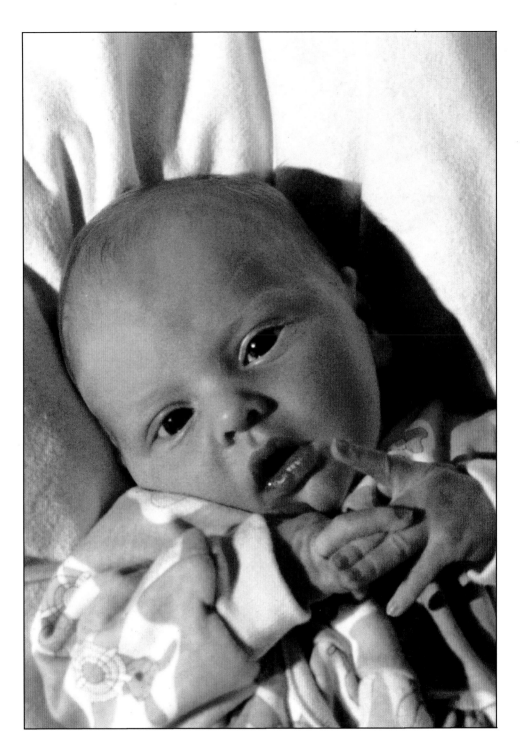

Elliot Gudgin at 1 month old

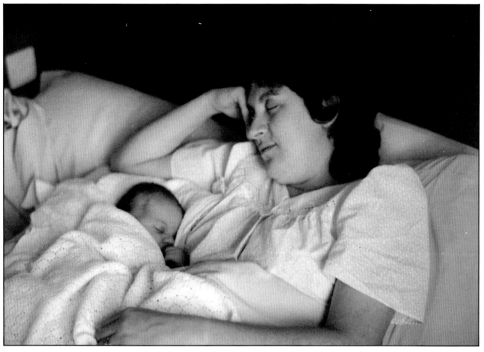

Yvonne Wheeler and Jamie

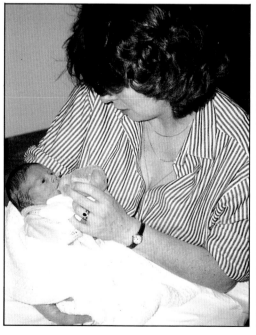

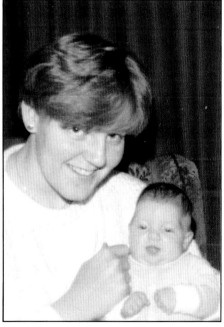

Josephine Dowd with Amy
at 6 weeks old

Linda Tuck with Harry

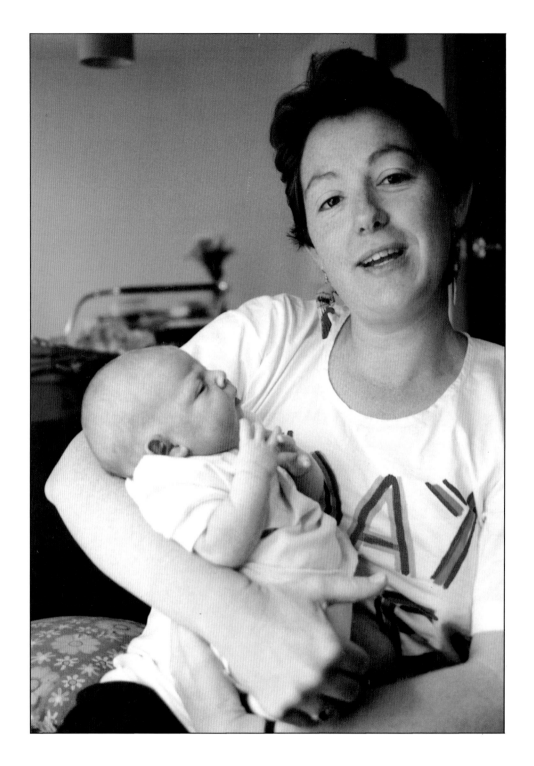

Ann Young with Madeleine at 17 days old

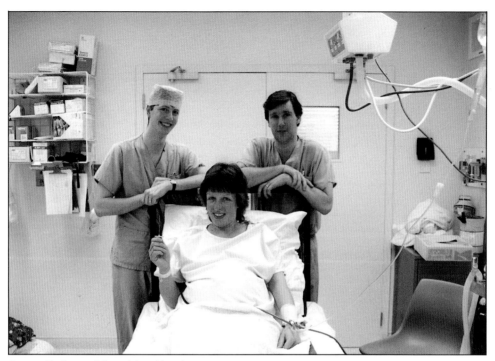

Serga Collett with epidural in place

Aren't I lucky . . . a little girl

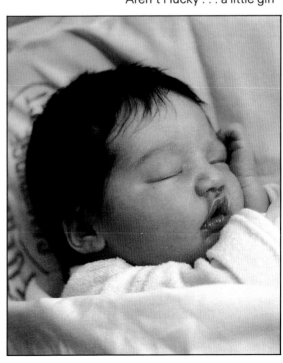

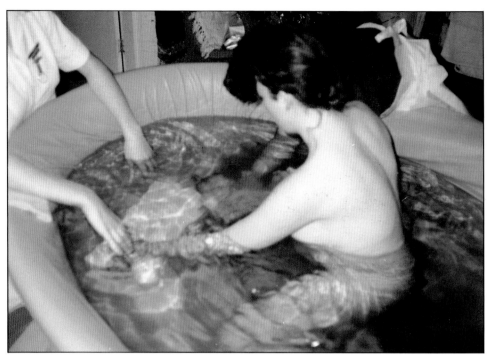

An underwater birth. Susan Jones with Shoshanna emerging underwater (*above*)

First breaths of air for Shoshanna (*below*)

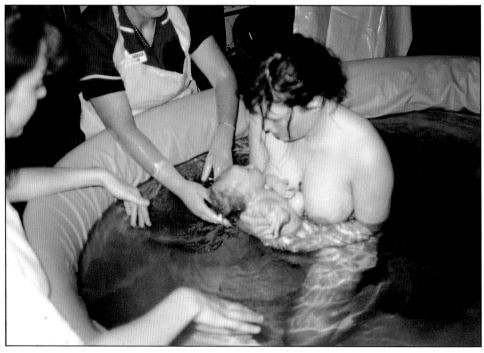

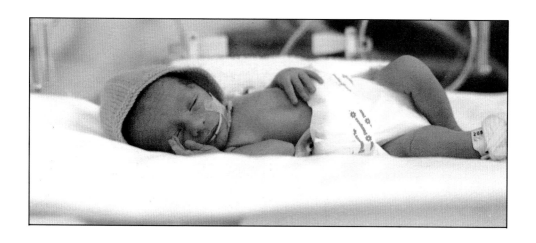

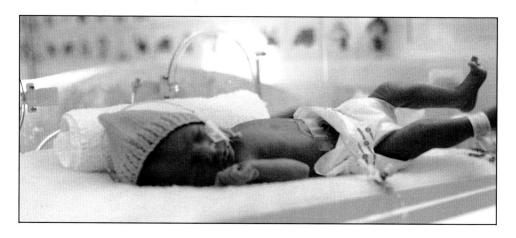

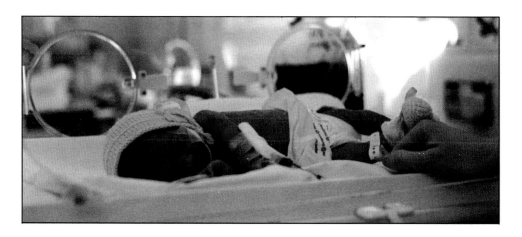

Sarah Marshall's triplets: from the top – Thomas, Edward and Louise

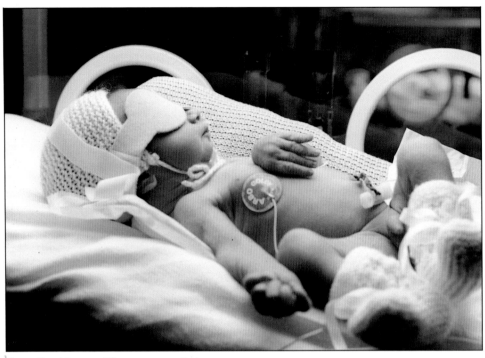

Jane Cook's son, Thomas, age 2 days

Martine Archer with Lewis (*centre*) and twins Jacob and Thymian (*below*)

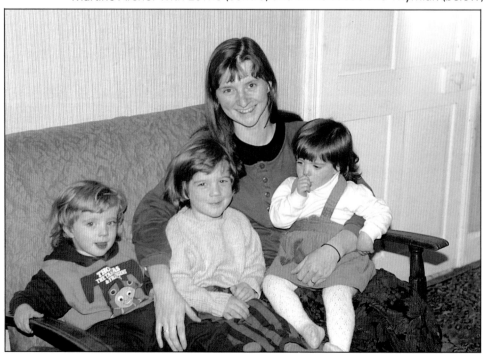

was reduced to tears – I wonder if they knew too. I suppose I'll never know.

When the triplets were two weeks old I went home without them. The arrangements were made and I was quite happy with the idea of coming into hospital every day to see them, but when it came to it, I didn't want to leave them, and once again I was reduced to a sobbing, gibbering idiot and despite the reassurance of the nurses I found this one of the hardest things I have ever had to do.

Not being allowed to drive at this stage, I was taken to the hospital at 8 o'clock each morning and collected at 7 or 8 o'clock each evening, so I was spending a great deal of time with the children, practically as much as if they were at home. Soon the day came when they were ready to come home. They were four weeks old. It was suggested that I should stay at hospital for one night and spend 24 hours caring for my babies so that I knew what things were really going to be like. The feeding routine had settled down, and things were pretty regimented, with each child feeding 20 minutes after the previous one had started. By this time, I had given up breast feeding as a bad job, I wasn't well enough equipped! Unfortunately, the night before my 24 hour shift, the night nurses had been thin on the ground, and all the babies in SCBU were fed when there was a spare moment, and our finely worked out routine went out of the window. I worked hard over the next 24 hours, only managing to get 45 minutes sleep in total. It seemed that the moment I managed to get to sleep the nurses were waking me again saying that a baby was crying and needed feeding – again. I wondered how anybody could expect me to cope at home, so I asked them to keep my offspring for another week, considering the results of the test-run and taking into account the fact that their father was going to be abroad anyway.

During the next week I began to feel so much better and more confident, and we finally took the babies home when they were exactly five weeks old on a snowy March day in 1986. There were many dark rings round eyes over the next weeks, months, years – there still are, but the help of a well adhered-to routine, and the fact that they slept from 11.00pm at night to 6.30am in the morning after only three weeks at home was the saving of me – and probably them! I would never have believed anything could be so dear to me.

See pictures page 131

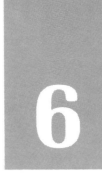

6

SPECIAL CARE BABIES

Many babies needing special care are premature and the reports in this section and in some other sections illustrate what marvellous care is provided by our special care baby units, and what tremendous things can be done for babies needing extra care. We have included one report of a full-term baby who needed special help because situations like this can often cause extra shock to the parents and is not always covered in books focusing on babies with extra needs. Having a special care baby is a joyful event tinged with fear and sadness for many parents with worries about growing too close to a baby when the future is uncertain. These reports are inspiring for parents who find themselves in similar situations.

It was 6.15pm on a quiet Sunday evening, seven weeks before the baby was due. My husband and stepson, both in the Parish church choir, were singing evensong and I was on my own and being very good resting on the sofa with my feet up watching television. There was a sudden wet sensation between my legs. My first thought was that I had been being remiss in doing my pelvic floor exercises and that I had wet myself. I gently eased myself off the sofa and across the hall to the cloakroom. There was suddenly a large puddle of water on the floor and I realised that this was fairly serious and that my waters had broken. I should at this juncture point out that the baby was not in the head down position, but lying diagonally across my stomach with his head tucked up under my ribs and feet down at the bottom. There was therefore no head to drop into place and seal the flow of water.

I telephoned my parents-in-law and my father-in-law went chasing off to fish Peter out of church and to wait for Jacob and to take charge of him. I telephoned the hospital and warned them of my imminent arrival and then I started to shake, and I didn't stop shaking until they gave me the anaesthetic in the operating theatre. Due to the baby's difficult position and the fact that I had had not a single contraction, Harry was born by Caesarean section at 9.36pm that evening. Peter had the first glimpse of him as he was rushed in to the Special Care Baby Unit (SCBU) across the corridor. He weighed 3lb 12oz and was put straight into an incubator and was given oxygen for the first few hours of his life. Luckily, his breathing was alright and he didn't need to be put on a ventilator. None of this I knew until much later when I came round from the operation and was taken upstairs to the ward. Peter had a polaroid picture of Harry in his incubator taken by the SCBU nurse for me. This is routine so that the baby's mother can see the baby if she is not well enough to go to see him herself.

I think it was at this point, 1 o'clock in the morning, that I really began to worry about Harry and whether he was going to live or die. I expected that at any moment a nurse would come into my room to tell me that Harry had died. Knowing a lot more now about premature babies that I did then, I realise that my fears were quite unfounded; 3lb 12oz is a very survivable weight especially as there were no other medical problems.

My first view of Harry was next morning. Having to go downstairs (admittedly in a wheelchair) in order to see him was a great incentive to overcoming the post-operative agony of a Caesarean and got me up and moving very quickly. All my fears came rushing back; he was absolutely tiny and looked so frail in his

LINDA TUCK

incubator. I was terrified of touching him; I thought he would break. He was breathing on his own without the aid of oxygen. The only intrusive extra was the thin plastic tube passed into his nose and taped to his cheek. Arriving at only 33 weeks Harry hadn't yet developed the instinct to suck, and the tube went directly into his stomach so that he could be fed easily and without exhausting himself. The nurse took him out of the incubator and put him in my arms for a first cuddle; such a tiny bundle.

Over the next day Harry moved up a nursery and we were taught how to change him in his incubator and to feed him through his tube. The four nurseries in the SCBU are graded from intensive care to almost ready to go home, and it is a great day for all parents when their baby moves up a nursery, a sure sign of progress. All parents are encouraged to participate as much as possible in the care of their babies. It was made very clear to me that while I was still in hospital myself, I was expected to get myself downstairs every three hours during the day to change and feed Harry. I did at least get to sleep through the nights.

Harry came home from the hospital when he was three weeks old and weighed $4^{1}/_{2}$lb. He thrived, and is now an extremely healthy, lively, almost five year old, about to start school. Looking back at the time five years ago, my main feelings now are that no-one said anything that prepared me for things going wrong, and that no-one reassured me enough immediately after his birth that everything was going to be well with Harry – maybe they didn't know!

The SCBU staff were wonderful, but too busy with the babies to give me as much time to talk as I needed and there was no other support staff.

My other strong feelings were that of failure that I hadn't had a natural birth and that, despite much effort, I had failed to breast-feed my son, often very difficult with a premature baby. Some help in dealing with these feelings would have been nice! In the end, a healthy happy baby is really all that matters.

See picture page 127

My labour began at lunchtime on 15th June a day before I was due. However, it was to be a very long labour. The contractions were very slow and niggling and like all first mothers I wondered if this really was labour. However, by 2.00am the next day I decided I needed to go to hospital, only to be told that I was only two centimetres dilated. I remember thinking when I arrived at the hospital that the next time I came out would be with a baby – how wrong could I be? After a distressing and painful night which I spent walking up and down and listening somewhat worriedly to other mothers giving birth, I was examined and sent home at 9.00am with two paracetamol and instructions to go to sleep. I was still only three centimetres dilated but the pains were every 10 minutes for one to two minutes. Sleep was out of the question and I was very distressed at being sent home after all my high hopes of the night before.

I paced, walked and dozed the whole of the next day with the pains continuing as before until early evening, when they gradually became more powerful and more frequent. However, by this time, I was scared to go back to hospital in case they sent me home again and thought me soft. However, having been unable to eat anything all day I decided I needed to go back to hospital again. At 9.00pm I had started to be sick with each contraction and was beginning to feel frightened and unsure of what to do.

When I arrived at hospital with my husband, who was by this time also very distressed and confused because we couldn't understand what was happening and why we couldn't do anything about it, the staff examined me and broke my waters telling me I was now eight centimetres dilated and 'it won't be too long now.' I was then given Pethidine and I can't remember much of the next few hours.

By 2.00am I needed more Pethidine and I was getting increasingly frightened and more and more tired, but the pains wouldn't let me sleep. At this point I was given the gas and air which I admit I used as a lifeline in what seemed to be an unbearably long process which was going nowhere.

The staff were very good but because I had been there so long; altogether there had been a few changeovers. I remember getting the overwhelming urge to push about 4.50am (having spent hours looking at the clock on the wall). It was a relief to want to push. I thought 'at last I can do something and get this over with'. I remember pushing and pushing for what seemed like hours without the aid of gas and air that had been taken away from me at this point. Nurses were shouting at me to 'try harder' and 'you're not doing it right' and 'the baby's stuck – it can't get round

SUSAN BARON

the bend'. This last terrified me but by now, after 31 hours of painful labour, I was too exhausted to do anything and I think I began to cry and sob as I was now convinced this would be the end of myself and the baby, but they assured me she was OK.

By 6.10am the nurses decided I needed a drip and forceps and I really think it was the sight of the forceps which made me push harder and finally, joy of joys the head was out and very quickly the rest of my daughter, but that was where the immediate joy ended. She wasn't breathing and was bright blue and quite honestly I thought she was dead. I remember thinking, 'my God, I've been through all that to get nothing at the end,' so before I had a chance to touch or bond with Rachel she was whisked away and given oxygen and then brought back to me for a very brief cuddle before being carted off to an incubator.

Nothing could detract from what I thought of as my beautiful daughter but by now as well as being scared I was also very angry. Why hadn't someone done something to speed the labour up? Why was I being punished by not having my baby with me? And what had I done that made this thing happen to us?

In due course I was wheeled through to see my baby with all the attendant wires, tubes and the bad headache they assured me she had, but all I could do was cry. My wonderful dream had all gone horribly wrong.

We weren't allowed to take Rachel out of the incubator for a cuddle for three days and I was terrified my child would grow up to be psychologically scarred because we hadn't had the bonding all the magazines say is so important. I discharged myself after three days and then made twice daily visits to the hospital for the next three weeks. How my husband coped at this time with a sick daughter and a mostly hysterical wife I don't know. He wasn't allowed to break down but had to keep cheerful for all of us. The staff on special care were fantastic and I couldn't have wished for better care and support for either Rachel or ourselves.

Three weeks later we were allowed to bring Rachel home. That was D-day when we started our life as a family. Rachel is now a bright, bubbly and perfect daughter but nothing will make me forget that time my hopeful bubble had been burst, and for a time was replaced with fear, distress and anguish. It was not the wonderful birth people talk about.

I was compelled to write the following account of my birth experience, not only because I would like to share it with others but also because I felt ill-prepared for the course of events and those who feel the same may find some encouragement in knowing what happened to me.

JANE COOK

My pregnancy was progressing well and I had remained fit and healthy with relatively few discomforts, so it was a surprise to me to experience a premature entry into labour at $34^1/_2$ weeks. An early spontaneous rupture of my membranes was the first thing that I felt unprepared for either by my antenatal classes or by the available literature.

I, like many, had pre-conceived ideas about how I would like my labour to be managed, but I had remained flexible in my approach to meet the needs of the situation. I spent much of the first stage of labour in one position. I had hoped to deal with this stage with massage and the adoption of various positions for comfort. However, I was greatly restricted both by the foetal monitor clipped to the baby's head (this had become necessary since the baby had shown signs of distress), and by the induction drip. Twenty eight hours had passed since my waters broke and I was showing no signs of having any spontaneous contractions. However, with a full understanding of why such procedures were necessary and with a great deal of support, I coped extremely well under the guidance of a superb midwife and excellent medical team. My labour was managed skilfully and sensitively and the delivery was a happy and relaxed experience.

Thomas had a very poor Apgar score at birth, was grey and limp and did not begin breathing for seven minutes. Immediately after delivery the cord was clamped and cut and he was taken to the resuscitation trolley in the corner of the delivery room. It was an anxious 10 minutes or so as the paediatricians tended to him, but I was able to hold him briefly before he was taken to the special care unit. During the third stage of labour my partner was taken to see him and it was wonderful for him to be able to come back and tell me of our son's progress.

Thomas was in an incubator, wired to machines to monitor his heart rate, respiration and temperature and had a drip for feeding and administering drugs. All these things were reassuringly explained by the staff of the unit and I was encouraged to visit and care for my baby both day and night as I wished. During the two and half weeks that Thomas was in special care I expressed milk for his feeds between attempts at breast and bottle feeding which he found difficult due to his prematurity.

My expectations of Thomas's birth were not fully realised. I was unable to experience that inital closeness, to hold him on my stomach and put him to the breast as I had hoped. Nor did I have the privilege to watch and admire him during the first few hours of his life. However, I am now able to recognise the positive aspects of having a 'special care' baby. During the early learning period when one is getting familiar with one's baby, I was given confidence by the expert help that was always to hand during such tasks as bathing and feeding. There were other distinct benefits too, such as several nights of adequate and undisturbed sleep.

I am happy to say that we now have with us a happy, beautiful, sociable, breast-feeding baby who is highly entertaining and rewarding.

In the knowledge that everything was done to deliver Thomas safely I am left with no sense of disappointment in not being able to follow a preferred birth plan. I learnt that a reasonable degree of flexibility and understanding are the main parts of what I feel is necessary to make your child's birth a treasured experience.

See picture page 132

7

POST-NATAL ISSUES

*Some of our reports covered problems most of
us have heard of, but fortunately few of us
experience. These didn't necessarily fit into
other categories. The small number of reports
chosen include the temporary hell of puerperal
psychosis which we are privileged to be able to
share, problems following suturing after
delivery, pre-eclampsia and one report where
the mother's extreme fitness concerned medical
staff. These are generally unusual problems and
most of us will remain unaffected by them.
Helpful contact numbers and addresses are at
the back of the book.*

SALLY RIGHTON

It is now some 12 weeks since the birth of our third daughter and I am now feeling quite settled and able to spare a little time to record the events of our labour experience and post-natal problems.

Of course, no-one really expects the arrival of their babies exactly on the 'expected date of delivery', and although I had been experiencing some rather strong irregular contractions during weeks 37–40, I didn't really expect that my labour would become established by the early hours of 10th May – the date I had been given by the doctor. After retiring to bed at about 11.30pm the previous evening, feeling decidedly uncomfortable and being aware of tightening, suddenly (about 12.15am) I felt my waters gushing gaily all over the bed in tune with an on-going contraction. My husband rushed to my rescue with a large towel. I thought it would be easier to stay put, instead of making more mess on the carpet! I was quite amazed, since with my two previous labours, my waters had not been broken until later. My first thought was to stay calm and try to cope with the now stronger contractions, that seemed to be coming at seven to ten minute intervals. But, in view of the fact that my second daughter had only taken two to three hours to arrive, we decided to arrange for a friend to come and sleep with our other children and get to the hospital as promptly as we could.

It was about 1.00am by the time we arrived at hospital, to be welcomed by the midwife at the door. We were admitted by a friendly nurse who took my antenatal details and other particulars. The midwife performed a routine examination and ran a foetal heart trace. We talked about pain relief and other practicalities, establishing a kind of rapport. I was managing to cope with these early contractions. They somehow didn't feel as dramatic as they had at home, possibly because we were getting excited, and now felt safe in capable hands.

In the next two hours I seemed to need endless trips to the toilet. I remained upright and fairly mobile. Pacing up and down and leaning over the bed from a sitting position on a hard supportive chair seemed to do the trick, and by about 3.30am I decided to use gas and air, as I was finding the increased strength of the pain very distracting. Having the mask to hold onto and grip tightly proved very successful. The pain seemed much worse when I had to lie down flat to be examined, but the midwife was quick and efficient and seemed quite happy with my progress so far.

It was very cosy, being together in the middle of the night. We managed a few laughs. The midwife was especially good at back massage. By now it was becoming exceedingly difficult to concentrate. We had no fixed ideas about the position to adopt for delivery and when the midwife came in to discuss it, we must have appeared very negative. I had no burning desire to remain standing, or to squat, but after finding the leaning position so helpful wondered at the possibility of an all-fours position. I was now starting to have a vague desire to push and the contractions were overwhelming. The midwife suggested we should transfer to the delivery room, where there would be space, and everything was to hand. So I walked to the delivery table and climbed aboard. I felt a tremendous contraction as I climbed up, ending in an all-fours fashion. I decided this was not right for me and changed to a half sitting position.

At first, I seemed to be holding back, allowing my body to do the work for me. But somehow I felt it would be more productive if I actually helped. Knowing that it would all soon be over, I gave three almighty pushes and the head was born. I remember feeling totally elated at this point, but didn't want to lose my concentration. It was now 4.20am and at last Nicola was born. We caressed her gently as she was lifted on to my tummy, so glad to notice that she appeared normal and very much like my first daughter.

After our joyful and delighted feelings had overwhelmed us, there followed a great sense of relief. I was able to enjoy the first moments with my new daughter with the peace of the dawn and the cosiness of that room. No-one rushed us, and I felt very emotional and moved by it all. The staff had been so kind and considerate and made it all seem very special. The placenta was safely delivered and Nicola was checked over and weighed. She was quite blue, apparently due to bruising from such a speedy entry into the world. No stitches were necessary!

The hospital is a small five-bedded unit with a separate isolation room. In no time at all I seemed to regain my strength and was rather disappointed that I was unable to return home after 48 hours. Firstly the doctor was concerned about Nicola's blueness and then shortly afterwards jaundice appeared and she lost a little too much weight, so insisted that my stay was lengthened. I had been longing to get back to my little family and I suppose I became rather selfishly agitated by the situation. I had originally wanted a home delivery, but this was not to be and unfortunately, because I had time in hospital to think, I can remember becoming inwardly apprehensive and doubtful about coping with a new baby and the demands of two active toddlers aged two and three.

My nights spent in hospital had been totally without sleep, and

I found myself very active during the day. I was finally discharged on the fifth day with diagnosed 'puerperal psychosis'. By that time I was almost oblivious to what was going on around me, although I was determined to act as normally as possible, in order to be discharged. I felt inwardly that I was becoming out of control and did not understand what was happening to me. The doctor suggested that perhaps I would overcome the psychosis at home in more relaxed surroundings but by the time I left hospital it was already too late. So much so, that later I imagined I had discharged myself and lived in fear of my doctor losing his job because of it.

I went home in the afternoon and my husband was aware that something was not quite right, even though no-one had told him about my problem. Firstly, I went into a frenzied, irrational state of panic and demanded that my elder daughters be sent next door for an hour or so, in order that I could try and calm down a bit. As the evening progressed, I felt myself slipping away, I couldn't concentrate at all. It was almost as if I had stepped outside of myself and someone else was carrying on with my actions. By the early hours of the morning I was uncontrollable and my husband could not restrain me. I was apparently abusive, delirious, confused and violent. I started to imagine all sorts of unlikely things. I even thought at one point that my husband was trying to kill me! In desperation, he telephoned the community midwife who came instantly and tried to help him. In turn the duty doctor was called. It was obvious that I needed help, so I was bundled off to a psychiatric hospital with Nicola. My husband and the midwife had insisted that Nicola should come with me, as they were anxious that I should continue breast-feeding, and I suppose they thought it would give me an extra incentive to get back to normality.

All I really remember are fragments of the following few weeks. I recall vividly the uncertainty in my husband's face as he left me in the middle of the dining room with an abundance of very odd people. I was afraid and totally frenzied. Things that seemed so very real to me were really my own imaginary dream. I felt as if my whole life was coming to an end and very strange. Conversations had double meanings, other patients became haunts from my past, the baby was a blur and I was now totally out of control. I could not communicate sensibly with anyone or anything. Initially sedation was necessary, to enable me to sleep. Then anti-depressants and tranquilizers were administered. I remember feeling highly suspicious of everyone. Electrical convulsive therapy followed, when I was finally persuaded to agree to it.

The staff were with me all the time, making sure that I fed the baby correctly and gradually helping me to look after her. The ward was not equipped for babies, it was for general patients with psychiatric illnesses. The baby literally slept in her carrycot on top of two chairs. Everything seemed difficult at first, but the staff had endless patience and I know the midwife was an enduring support.

After the third ECT treatment, a marked difference occurred in my behaviour, as if I was slowly awakening from a bad dream. I was now sleeping at night (being woken for night feeds), and beginning to slowly take an interest in my surroundings, the baby and other patients. I felt very depressed and could not comprehend what was happening to me, but tried desperately to think of nice things to keep me sane. Picking up the pieces was not an easy process, I felt selfish and guilty at first, and I began to worry if the children would be marred by this ordeal.

As it was, friends locally rallied around and had helped at home, and much love and concern was shown by friends and relations alike. The support was tremendous and I will remember the warmth of friends, when we were so very much in need of them, for the rest of my life. On reflection, I am shattered by the whole experience but grateful that its severity passed within a few weeks. Other mothers who suffer from this problem can take months and even years to recover. Gradually, with the help of drugs I have been able to return to a level of normality (what is normal?). I still feel a shadow of my former self. Pulling myself together after having sunk so low has not been easy for me. I am usually a happy and reasonably well-balanced person, although sometimes prone to behaving impulsively and frantically, as most people probably are. It is only now that I am beginning to enjoy Nicola, who has been a lovely and perfect little soul since her arrival. I thank God for my healthy daughters.

GAYNOR

I got pregnant whilst living in Holland with my Dutch husband and I had my baby there too. I had a lovely pregnancy except for the last few weeks when I had several niggly problems. I'm of a very small build, take size three shoes and normally weigh 7st, so I was very anxious that I was not going to be big enough to part with my baby. The midwife paid no attention to my worries and scoffed at my enquiries over pain killers; in Holland they don't even have gas and air and most women prefer to give birth at home. In the end she said I could have Pethidine if I needed it.

My baby was five weeks premature. I was not initially afraid at the first signs of labour, just very excited. I first had a 'show' then a few hours later had regular contractions. I coped with this for several hours then when my midwife came to check on me at midnight I asked about painkillers (I'd been in labour since around 3.30pm but my contractions had been bearable). 'Not yet,' she said, and said she'd be back around 3.00am. I was getting nervous and said I'd be better off in hospital. We had to go by taxi as we had no car. We'd only just got into the 'panting' room when my waters broke. I thought I'd had it and looked around expecting to see this baby. By this time the midwife had still not arrived. It was about 12.30am and I wanted to push. They kept asking me if I really wanted to push or was it that I needed to go to the toilet, and I hadn't a clue – it felt like the worst constipation ever.

They quickly wheeled me into the 'action' room and I'd barely rolled onto the delivery bed when I started to feel like I'd lost complete control of my body. The midwife ran in to tell me his head was almost visible and not to push yet. I was trying to remember that silly breathing and hyperventilated – all my face and arms got pins and needles. I began to get hysterical and begged for a painkiller only to be told it was too late. Why oh why didn't they tell me you had to have Pethidine much earlier?

I never expected such powerful contractions. She was telling me not to push but my whole body was just heaving and contracting; I had no power over it and started making these awful animal noises and howls. I also didn't realise that the head would keep slipping back up several times and this really worried me. I expected that once I saw the head it would come out all at once (I had a mirror), but I was more worried about my anus which was swollen and purple. The midwife yelled at me to stop screaming and then to my horror started to stab around my vagina with a huge needle attached to a ten millilitre syringe full of local anaesthetic. I realised I was about to receive the dreaded episiotomy.

I kicked the syringe through the air totally distressed by this point and was horrified when she grabbed the scissors and attempted to snip me without any local anaesthetic. Nurses were holding me down; my husband was a nervous wreck and I was kicking and wriggling for all I was worth. She told me not to push if I'd no contractions – by that time my contractions had completely stopped which I'm sure was stress related, but I was determined to get that baby out without her cutting me, so I pushed with all my might and out he came. I tore slightly so after touching my child for a few seconds he was whisked away to an incubator at the other side of the hospital and I was sprayed with a bit of local anaesthetic (she may as well have put salt on it), and appallingly stitched up. I was allergic to the stitches and they said I needed to be re-stitched which gave me so much scar tissue I still can't make love properly almost 18 months later. I felt I was never allowed to bond with my son properly. I failed miserably at breastfeeding and for the 12 days I was in hospital I was made to feel totally inadequate.

The baby and I are very close now so I can't say the traumatic birth had any long term effects on our relationship, but it has definitely changed my marriage as I'm now scared of sex and of pain in any form. I think I could have had a very positive birth had I been in England with sympathetic people, and I'm still very bitter about the whole thing.

TINA
STECKLES

I approached the birth of my first child without any previous knowledge or experience of childbirth, no friends or sisters to give me a clue. I did, however, have complete confidence that the hospital would take good care of me. I'd just spent 12 years working as an occupational therapist in hospitals all over the country (not in obstetrics, unfortunately), so felt familiar and very comfortable in a hospital environment. This state did not persist for very much longer.

I was admitted two weeks after my expected delivery date, to be induced, spending the night before the procedure (whatever it was), was to be carried out in sleepless anxiety and feeling a failure: i.e. unable to deliver on time. I was then given an enema, the first of many things that I would have 'done to me'. Later I was shown into a small 'operating room', very clinical, and left alone for approximately one hour. No one came to reassure me and I began to feel that I'd been forgotten. I began to feel panicky and totally out of control of the situation. Nothing in the books I'd read or anything I'd been told by antenatal staff prepared me for a baby reluctant to make an entrance of its own accord.

Finally, a nurse appeared and strapped me up to have waters broken; later wires were attached to the baby's head and I was given two lots of something to start my contractions, the first lot not having worked. I had told my husband that I'd telephone him when I was actually in labour but wasn't quite sure when I'd have the opportunity to get to a telephone. I had imagined walking round, talking to people, reading my book, listening to tapes whilst in labour, but I was now destined to remain flat on my back for the next 36 hours. The severity of pain was so unexpected I could only concentrate on trying to cope with the increasingly strong contractions using relaxation techniques in between and praying that I wouldn't scream out or panic. I asked a nurse to contact my husband and then settled down to 'hard labour'. Using the skills I'd learned from transcendental meditation, I managed to cope with every wave of painful contractions and when a nurse asked if I'd like something for the pain, I accepted gladly without even asking what I was being injected with.

My husband had arrived and was surprised that I kept falling asleep in between contractions. I'd had Pethidine and later had a 'top up'. At this stage I was not aware of any in between stages, just contractions coming fast, but still tried to maintain a calm state although I was getting tired and disorientated. When the doctor asked me in a brisk manner 'did I play a lot of squash?', I simply did not understand the implication of his question. I answered 'no, I'd never played squash in my life'. He then asked whether I played a lot of sport. No, I didn't participate in any games whatsoever. If he'd told me that my pulse rate had dropped to 50, I would have told him, 'so what?' I'd once got it down to 43 after a particularly deep meditative experience – all through pregnancy I had daily meditated to benefit both myself and baby. Keeping my blood pressure down, etc. – so I believed.

Things happened with great speed at this stage. Three cardiac team doctors rushed in with portable equipment, attached monitors to my chest and followed everyone else into the delivery room along with my trolley-bed. I was given a large episiotomy to facilitate the snatched delivery of my baby. I felt as though he'd been ruthlessly dragged out of me and I was very upset to see the forceps marks on his poor little face. His head looked bullet shaped. He was rushed away to the nursery. It was felt that my heart rate needed further monitoring, to be on the safe side, for a further 24 hours during which time I was unable to leave my bed, having wires and monitors attached to me. I wasn't able to see my baby at all during this time. I felt desolate.

I had been badly bruised during the delivery and suffered retention of urine, the nerves having been bruised – I wasn't able to empty my bladder independently. I felt like an old woman as I was catheterised manually by the nurse, strapped up to a machine and feeling more like the victim of a road accident rather than an ecstatic new mum. I began to feel very resentful and terribly disappointed. I had expected to hold my baby and feel proud and happy; instead I felt like a post-operative patient and to my interminable shame I blamed my baby for my predicament. I'll never get over the guilt of this. No one has ever said the monitoring of my heart either revealed a health risk or showed me as fit. I was given a six week follow-up appointment which involved an exercise stress test which showed no abnormality. I had spent the previous six weeks believing that I could have a problem, wondering if I would have much longer to live and see my child grow up. I remain extremely fit and healthy but wish my labour had been handled more sensitively and had been less traumatic.

A HAPPY ENDING

Gestation times – books versus babies

Since Dawn and I began work on this book I have conceived, miscarried, conceived again and three days ago Angus Montgomery Stewart was safely delivered. The book is, meanwhile, staggering towards the end of its gestation period – and we hope it will arrive in the world as easily.

At 32 weeks I noticed signs of impending labour – previous experiences told all my instincts that the baby was getting ready to show its face. At my antenatal appointment I 'warned' my GP that I didn't think I could hold on too long. I had optimistically opted for a home delivery, and he repeated his previous diatribe about having to go to 37 weeks in order to be allowed to stay at home. He also advised me that it would make a big difference to the baby if I could wait until at least 34 weeks.

But how do you wait? Short of being stitched up, nobody had any real suggestions – rest might help, but there were no guarantees, and rest just makes me stressed, so on the whole I decided stress-avoidance was advisable and I just hoped for the best.

One day short of 33 weeks, I felt a strong uterine cramp and raced upstairs to pack a bag. Nothing followed, but I know my own body, and I cancelled plans for the following day. Sure enough, by midnight the contractions were very mild, but regular. I warned Adrian not to sleep too deeply and set about reading my book of childrens names (there's nothing quite like being prepared!).

My previous delivery, a girl now two years old, had developed extremely rapidly, so although contractions were still mild, I telephoned the hospital who said that at 33 weeks I must come straight in. So, in we went. We were welcomed warmly by a midwife who 'left us to it'. Things continued to develop slowly but nicely, and this labour was so similar to my son's, six years ago, that I knew, without a doubt, that this was another boy.

By 6.30am an internal showed me to be eight to nine centimetres dilated. The pain was still minimal, and I was calm and happy. Unfortunately, a paediatrician then arrived and was insistent that the dangers of foetal distress at 33 weeks were such that

I must be strapped down with monitors. I wasn't happy, but I was persuaded that the baby's health came first, so I reluctantly climbed onto the bed and lay flat. The baby was fine and strong, but all contractions stopped. I was frustrated, and stayed that way until lunch time – flat on my back and going nowhere!

At 1.00pm the shift changed and I talked my frustrations through with a new midwife who jogged my memory back to a tip taught at NCT classes – nipple stimulation!

She left me alone, I rolled my nipples mercilessly and it worked like magic! Within 10 minutes the contractions were coming thick and fast. I begged to be mobilised, and the wonderful midwife allowed me on the floor with a beanbag, as long as I kept the foetal monitor on.

From then on it was plain sailing. I breathed through the pain, feeling the contractions to be ever-more productive.

By 3.00pm I was ready to push. The midwife, who cannot be praised highly enough, didn't bother me with an internal assessment but trusted me to know myself. I waited until it felt just right and pushed. The baby's head came into sight, and the second and third pushes delivered him, still in his amniotic sac – my second 'dry' baby! He punctured the sac with one angry kick and let out a loud shout. Angus weighed in safely at 5lb 13oz. Five minutes later the placenta followed naturally, and within another five minutes I was washed, dressed and ready to run a marathon. I have never felt so well and happy.

ENDPIECE

This book should be of great interest to expectant parents who hope to read a little more about birth. We hope that the joy experienced by most parents inspires them to transcend the fears engendered by the stories of difficult childbirth but make no apology for including these. Some women *do* have Caesareans and some women *do* have forceps deliveries and so on and are here to tell the tale!

We hope that men will want to read these stories which come mainly from women to help them to understand what giving birth is like from a female perspective. Most of all we hope that professionals who are involved with the management of labour and aftercare, the obstetricians, midwives, GPs, nursing staff and health visitors are able to empathise with the parents in these accounts and to realise their own importance in helping to create a positive experience of childbirth for women, even in stressful conditions. While many accounts praised the staff involved with their deliveries, others encountered unhelpful attitudes or responses which they interpreted as such during labour.

The management of labour is going through great changes as practices alter and as parents become slowly more assertive and knowledgeable. This book gives a chance to 'put oneself in the role of the other' and to learn from the experiences as written by parents in their own words.

HELPFUL ADDRESSES

Below is a list of addresses of organisations which readers may find useful. They include support groups for parents and also groups involved in choice in childbirth.

Active Birth Centre
55 Dartmouth Park Road
London NW5 1SL
Tel: 071-267 3006
Offers ante-natal classes, post-natal support, teachers and birth pool hire, etc.

Association for Postnatal Illness
25 Jerdan Place
Fulham
London SW6 1BE
Tel: 071-386 0868

Association of Radical Midwives
The Coppice
62 Greetby Hill
Ormskirk L39 2DT
Tel: 0695 572776
Supports those experiencing difficulty in giving/receiving good maternity care.

Baby Life Support Systems
(BLISS)
17–21 Emerald Street
London WC1N 3QL
Tel: 071-831 9393
Through BLISSLINK offers support to families of special care babies.

British Acupuncture Association
and Register
34 Alderney Street
London SW1V 4EV
Tel: 071-834 1012
Publishes register and yearbook of acupuncturists.

British Meditation Society
51 Aldridge Road Villas
London W11

British Homeopathic Association
27a Devonshire Street
London W1N 1RJ
Tel: 071-935 2163
Primarily for lay people, offering books and documentation, including lists of homeopathic doctors, hospitals and chemists.

British Pregnancy Advisory
Service
Austy Manor
Wooton Wawen
Solihull
West Midlands B95 6BX
Tel: 0564 793225
Referral service with information about clinics in other areas.

Caesarean Support Network
2 Hurst Park Drive
Huyton
Liverpool L39 1TF
Tel: 051-480 1184
Sadly, we do not know of a support network for forceps and other operative procedures.

Centre of Advice on Natural
Alternatives
Tyddyn Y Mynydd
Llanelli Hill
Abergavenny
Gwent NP7 0PN

Cervical Stitch Network
Fairfield
Woolverton Road
Norton Lindsey
CV35 8LA
Advice & information regarding cervical suture during pregnancy.

Episiotomy Support Group
232 Ifield Road
West Green
Crawley
Sussex RH11 7HY
Tel: 0293 540416
For women who have experienced episiotomies.

Foundation for the Study of
Infant Deaths
35 Belgrave Square
London SW1X 8QB
Tel: 071-235 0965
Helpline (24 hrs) 071-235 1721
Support for bereaved families of cot death infants.

Home Birth Centre
Flat 3
55 Elm Grove
Southsea
Hampshire PO5 1JF
Tel: 0705 864494

Hysterectomy Support Network
The Venture
Green Lane
Upton
Huntingdon PE17 5YE
Tel: 081-690 5987

Issue (Infertility issues)
Birmingham Settlement
318 Summer Lane
Birmingham B19 3RL
Tel: 021-359 4887
Helpline 021-359 7359

La Leche League
BM 3424
London WC1N 6XX
Tel: 071-404 5011
071-242 1278 (24 hours).
Help with breastfeeding

Maternity Alliance
15 Britannia Street
London WC1X 9JP
Tel: 071-837 1265
*An independent national
organisation campaining for
improvements in rights and
services for mothers.*

Miscarriage Association
c/o Clayton Hospital
Northgate
Wakefield WF1 3JS
Tel: 0924 200799

National Childbirth Trust
Alexandra House
Oldham Terrace
London W3 6NH
Tel: 081-992 8637

Pre-eclamptic Toxaemia Society
17 South Avenue
Hullbridge
Essex SS5 6HA
Tel: 0702 232533

Pre-eclampsia Society
c/o Dawn James
Ty Lago
Carmel
Caernarvon
Gwynedd
Tel: 0286 880057

Pre-Natal Therapy Association
14 Edgar Road
Winchester
Hanmpshire
*Seminars & lectures on
manipulation and massage to
relieve pre birth traumas.*

SANDS (Stillbirth and Neonatal
Death Society)
28 Portland Place
London W1N 4DE
Tel: 071-436 5881

Shiatsu Society
14 Oakdene Road
Redhill
Surrey RH1 6BT
Tel: 0737 767896

Society to Support Home
Confinements
Lydgate
Lydgate Lane
Wolsingham DL13 3HA
Tel: 0388 528044

Support After Termination for
Abnormality (SAFTA)
29/30 Soho Square
London W1V 6JB
Tel: 071-439 6124

Twins & Multiple Births
Association (TAMBA)
59 Sunnyside
Worksop
Nottinghamshire S81 7LN

Waterbabies (birth pool hire)
c/o Annette Gaskell
874 Burnley Road
Walmersley
Bury
Lancashire
Tel: 061-764 2616